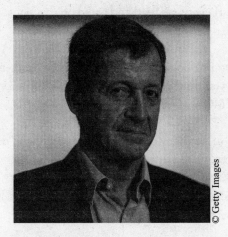

© Getty Images

Alastair Campbell is best known for his role as Tony Blair's chief spokesman and strategist. He has written several best-selling books, including *The Blair Years, Winners* and *All in the Mind*. A former 'Mind Champion of the Year', he is an ambassador for several mental health charities. In November 2017 he was awarded an honorary fellowship of the Royal College of Psychiatrists in recognition of his role in breaking down the stigma surrounding mental illness.

'Supremely readable, supremely useful. Unflinching, clear-eyed, honest, raw and revealing, this book may be the most important achievement of Alastair Campbell's vivid and varied life . . . *Living Better* is indispensable' STEPHEN FRY

'Fascinating, compelling and totally relatable. There were times it moved me to tears, other times it had me smiling and laughing, but above all it made me reflect that I am not alone . . . If everyone read and acted on this book, the world would be a better place' DENISE WELCH

'An astounding book, pacy and full of good concrete ideas . . . at times, very funny. I feel I understand depression so much better' SIMON MAYO

'Helpful to so many people, people who have depression, and people who love them' SUSANNAH REID

'Profound and moving . . . everyone should read it' JOHANN HARI, author of *Lost Connections*

'It is fascinating to see how someone seen as strong and tough can talk so openly about his vulnerabilities' MARO ITOJE, Saracens and England rugby-player

'Part deeply personal memoir, part self-help book, but above all a love letter to his family, and especially to Fiona, his partner of 40 years' *Libération* (France)

'Deeply honest . . . [Campbell] articulately reflects on these issues in sharp detail, creating an all-encompassing and intricate look into mental health' *The i*

'Deeply honest and all-encompassing, *Living Better* will strike a chord with almost all of us' *Irish News*

Living Better

HOW I LEARNED TO
SURVIVE DEPRESSION

Alastair Campbell

JOHN MURRAY

For F, F and F

First published in Great Britain in 2020 by John Murray (Publishers)
An Hachette UK company

This paperback edition published in 2021

2

A CIP catalogue record for this title is available from the British Library

Paperback ISBN 978-1-529-33183-7
eBook ISBN 978-1-529-33184-4

Typeset in Simoncini Garamond by Hewer Text UK Ltd, Edinburgh
Printed and bound in Great Britain by Clays Ltd, Elcograf S.p.A.

John Murray policy is to use papers that are natural, renewable
and recyclable products and made from wood grown in sustainable
forests. The logging and manufacturing processes are expected to
conform to the environmental regulations of the country of origin.

John Murray (Publishers)
Carmelite House
50 Victoria Embankment
London EC4Y 0DZ

www.johnmurraypress.co.uk

CONTENTS

Part II:
My Search For a Cure

PREFACE

On a dark Sunday night last winter, I almost killed myself. Almost. I've had a lot of almosts. Never gone from almost to deed. Don't think I ever will. But it was a bad almost. Bad. That I didn't go through with it had a lot to do with a jam jar.

It's a long story. I'll start at the beginning.

I

ME, MY LIFE,
MY DEPRESSION

1

MY CHILDHOOD, MY FAMILY

On the face of it, I have it all. A wonderful partner with whom I have shared forty years of my life. Three amazing children who make me incredibly proud to be their dad. I have great friends. A nice home. A dog I love and who loves me even more. Money is not a problem. I have had several satisfying careers, first as a journalist, then in politics and government. Now I get paid to tour the world and tell audiences what I think. I have the freedom to campaign for the causes I believe in, something not always present in my previous two careers: as a journalist I was dependent on events; in politics, I had to subsume my life into the needs and demands of others. With today's freedom, I can pick and choose, and I do. So when I decided to write this book, for example, I did just that, and pushed other things into the background. Because I can.

But there is one major part of my life that I cannot control. Depression. It is a bastard; despite all my good luck and opportunities, all the things that should ensure I am happy and fulfilled, it keeps coming. This book is an attempt to explain my depression, to explore it, to make sense of it, properly to understand it – where it may have come from, why it keeps coming and what, if anything, I can do to live a better life despite it.

In doing so, I hope to be able to find answers that may help me, and that my story and the telling of it may help others too. We all know someone with depression. There is barely a family untouched by it. We may be talking about it more than we did, back in the era of 'big boys don't cry' – they did, you know – when a 'brave face' or a 'stiff upper lip' or a 'best foot forward' was seen as the only way to go. But we still don't talk about it enough. There is still stigma, shame and taboo. There is still the feeling that admitting to being sad or anxious, let alone chronically depressed, makes us weak. It took me years, decades even, to get to this point, but I now passionately believe that the reverse is true and that speaking honestly about our feelings and experiences (whether as a depressive or as the friend or relative of a depressive) is the first and best step on the road to recovery. So that is what I am trying to do here.

To begin with, I want to go right back to the start, to my birth, my family and the broadly happy childhood which followed.

Once there were six of us. And now we are just two.

We were a family of exiles: an intensely Scottish family living in England. My Dad, Donald Campbell, was a crofter's son born on the Hebridean island of

Tiree in 1922. My mother Betty, four years younger, was the daughter of an Ayrshire farmer. They met when my Dad, then a student vet at Glasgow University, was visiting the farm where she grew up. Once they got engaged, the marriage almost never happened, because my Dad insisted he would never leave Scotland. My Mum called off the engagement and headed south herself, to work in a London hotel; eventually he followed, first working in Hampshire, then as a full partner in practice with fellow Scot, Murdo Ferguson, in Keighley in the James Herriot territory of Yorkshire. That was where we four children were all born, in Victoria Hospital. I was the third boy in a row, born on 25 May 1957. My sister Elizabeth, born two years later, owes her life to the fact that my mother was determined to keep going till she had a daughter. Had I been a girl we would have been five not six.

That we are now just two, me and Liz, is because our older brothers Donald and Graeme died prematurely. They were both aged sixty-two. Which is, worryingly enough, my age right now.

I was closest in age to Graeme, who was born just thirteen months before me, and for long periods of our childhood we were inseparable. Considering that we spent most of our upbringing sharing a bedroom, and had a shared passion for sport and, later, languages, I often think we should have been closer as adults. He was clever, funny, but never made the most of his undoubted talents. He had next to no interest in wealth, material comfort or making a good career.

Of the four of us, he was the least enamoured of our Scottish identity. Donald and I both took up Dad's offer to teach us to play the bagpipes. Graeme refused, referring to our chosen instrument, which required considerable time devoted to practice, simply by the anagram – 'gabsepip!' And while Donald and I felt no embarrassment, and even a certain pride, in dressing up in a kilt, Graeme made so clear his objection to being asked to 'wear a skirt' that before long, Mum and Dad gave up trying to persuade him.

He dropped out of his first university, though did OK at the next one, then went off to America one day for a short trip and didn't come back for years. When Donald visited him once, he was shocked at the squalor he lived in, with a mattress, a sleeping bag and not much else. He lived for a while in Poland, mainly teaching English, and there he met his wife, Ania, and they had a son, Mike. The marriage failed, not least because of his drinking, and though he improved on the father front in later years, by then the damage to his health caused by decades of heavy smoking, drinking and a peripatetic lifestyle meant he didn't have long left to go.

He had resilience though. Shortly before he went into the operating theatre to have both his legs removed – 'one for the booze, one for the fags', as he wryly accepted – the doctor told him in front of Liz and me: 'I do need to warn you that you may be entering the final stages of your life.' In other words, the last few moments before the general anaesthetic took hold might well be his last moments of conscious life.

'I understand,' he said, quietly, to the doctor, then looked up at Liz and me with a sense of regret but also resignation in his eyes.

'You'll be fine,' I said, not really believing it.

Liz and I walked alongside him, a hand apiece on his bony shoulders, as he was wheeled to the operating theatre, and only as he disappeared through the double doors did we let our emotion at the enormity of what was happening pour out, hugging each other, both in tears now, Liz saying: 'I don't think he will come out again.'

Neither of us expected him to survive. That he did, and went on to live for several more years, spoke to that resilience but also, I think, to his desire to make amends to Mike. For a while, once he was out of hospital, Graeme and Mike lived together in Retford. It was not easy for either of them – and eventually Graeme had to move into a nursing home – but at least he was trying.

Graeme knew he was far from a perfect husband, or perfect dad. He knew that Mike had had to see his father in a state no child should have to see a parent. Mike knew something was wrong in their relationship. So did Graeme. But he was never great at facing up to difficult things. He hoped they would go away on their own, without him having to decide or do the things he needed to fix them, perpetually putting them off until another day. Whereas 'get a grip . . . let's sort this . . . can we please do something' are among my mantras, 'later . . . we'll see . . . it'll work out' were among Graeme's.

His final days were reminiscent of when our Dad died. Just as Dad had waited to see all of us before finally he gave up the fight, so I think Graeme was determined to see Mike one last time before bowing to the inevitable. Dad had been ill for some months. Liz, Donald and I had seen him, talked to him, hoping we said what we needed to say, and he needed to hear. At the time Graeme was living in Poland. He and Dad had never been particularly close, and Graeme perhaps resented that Dad used to refer to him as 'my English son'. But Dad hung on until he travelled back to see him so that they could say goodbye. When Dad finally died a few days later, alone of the four of us, Graeme did not want to see the body at the funeral directors. I tried to persuade him it was an important moment of closure, but he was adamant that he would find it too upsetting.

It was clear that Graeme's life really was now in its final stages, and he had given instructions that he wanted no more drugs, no more pain. Mike, who was working a couple of hours away, called to say he was coming to see him tomorrow. The phone call was their final proper conversation and the last words Graeme said to his son, barely audible but clear enough, were 'I love you'. By the time Mike got there the next day, Graeme was struggling for breath and struggling to speak, but was at least able to sit with his son for a long time. It was the last day of his life. Later that night the home called to say he had gone.

I think Graeme had similar issues with depression and addiction to mine. I can't help feeling if he had confronted them he would still be here. But how deep must the addictive and self-destructive instinct run when you can remove an oxygen mask and drag your legless body from bed to wheelchair so you can head outside into the freezing cold just to gasp down a few drags of a cigarette.

It was when I witnessed that, at the care home where eventually he died, that I realised there was no point nagging him about his smoking any more. He had chosen his path. By then he weighed less than half what he used to. And when he went – that night after not just Mike but some of our favourite cousins from Scotland had come to see him – I had an overwhelming feeling of sadness, but also thought how could two people with the same parents and upbringing, with so many similarities, end up taking such different paths? Then again, looking at so many other families, maybe that is not odd at all.

When we got the call to say he had finally passed away, Mike and I went to see the body, and Mike, through his tears, said something very wise: 'He didn't have a perfect life. But he did live. He travelled. He learned languages. He had passions. He had knowledge. He was a good man who made some bad choices. He was a clever man who didn't always use his cleverness well.'

Donald, three years older than me, was a very different story. Outward-going, a people pleaser, a socialiser, he loved to talk, to anyone, about anything, apart from politics, sport and, until later in life when he became a firm believer in 'the Big Man Upstairs', religion. He lived in Glasgow for most of his life, and hated with a passion the sectarian element of the Celtic–Rangers football rivalry. Because he spent so much of his life in Scotland, he had a different accent to the rest of us. When he once appeared with me in a TV programme about bagpipes, I'm sure many viewers wondered how the two of us could be brothers. But if the small gap in age meant I was closer to Graeme in early childhood, Donald and I always got on, and our childhood closeness was cemented in adulthood by his mental illness. It was so severe there was no way – as Graeme did and as perhaps I did too in my depression-drowning drinking days – of avoiding having to confront it. Donald's illness is the real reason that I became passionate about the issue of mental health.

For both of us growing up in our very Scottish home, albeit in West Yorkshire, Scottish culture was always a big part of our lives. When Dad taught us to play the bagpipes from a young age, Donald, the least academically minded of the four of us, was determined to make a career out of his natural talent for pipe music. So he joined the Scots Guards, less to fight wars than to play music. He did his share of fighting, in Northern Ireland especially, but his military career came to an abrupt end one night in the summer of 1976. My mother said her life changed with the phone call that came that night 'and it never changed back again'.

The family was by then living in Leicester. I was between school and university. The call from the Ministry of Defence told us that Donald had been taken to hospital. No, he was not injured, but had had some kind of breakdown, and had been taken first to Woolwich hospital, then to the military psychiatric hospital in Netley, near Southampton. His fellow Guardsman Kevin Budd, who remained a lifelong friend and whose wife Karin visited Donald regularly, later described it as feeling as though Donald had been 'frozen in time', unable to connect with the world around him. Mum got hold of Dad, and he and I set off south. The Donald we saw several worried, silent hours later was not the Donald we had seen a few weeks earlier when he was home on leave, splashing out cash to Graeme, me and Liz. Perhaps that was one of the reasons we never saw it coming. The money he gave out, loving having a salary for the first time, felt like evidence that 'he's enjoying it, he's happy, he's loving his job, he's loving playing the pipes in the Scots Guards'. So we didn't see it coming at all.

And now . . . there was a childlike fear in his eyes, and nonsense coming from his mouth. He had drawn an immaculate, elaborate cross on the wall, an outline of Jesus upon it, and kept pointing to it, saying 'he knows, you know'.

Though my Dad was a vet, and therefore trained in scientific thinking, he knew little about the illness we were now told Donald had. Schizophrenia. I knew even less. But from that moment it became a huge part of our lives.

After Donald's death, my sister and I put together a little map as we counted up all the different hospitals in which he had been treated. It ran the length of Britain, from Netley in the deep south, where it all started, through London, Leicester in the Midlands, Hull in the north, various wonderful places around Scotland, and finally Kingsmill in Mansfield, where he died.

Schizophrenia is a truly horrible illness. You can't see it. No crutches. No sudden baldness. No bandages. No scars. It is all in the mind. People who have it often become pariahs, shunned in the workplace, derided and abused on the streets. I wish people wouldn't use that cliché 'split personality'; it's as awful as the way people use the word 'schizophrenic' when they mean there are two views of something, or that someone has good moods and bad. It minimises. It misunderstands. It stigmatises. Schizophrenia is a severe *illness* in which the workings of your mind become separated from the reality around you. And it can be terrifying.

Imagine a cacophony of voices in your head, screaming, telling you to do things you *normally* know you shouldn't. Then imagine plugs, sockets and light switches, road signs and shop signs, talking to you. Imagine sitting in a public place busy with people going about their business and thinking every single word being thought by everyone is about *you*. Imagine watching TV and being sure everyone is talking about you. And then imagine snakes coming out of the floor and wild cats charging through the walls and ceilings. Donald had all that and more when he was in crisis.

So, imagine the strength of character it takes to deal with that in a way that led so many people to love him so much, not out of sympathy – he didn't want sympathy – but out of an appreciation of the real him, unclouded by illness. That is an achievement of epic proportions. Doctors and medication played a big role in this achievement, but he himself played the biggest part.

Also imagine having all that to deal with and never saying 'it's not fair'. I said it, for more than forty years, from the first day Dad and I saw him lying in that bed, terrified. 'Not fair. Why Donald?' I said it, often. He didn't. Not then. Not ever. Not once.

Imagine being so keen to be a soldier, making it, doing well but then due to this illness his career terminating at a stroke, the prestige of playing in the Scots Guards' 1st Battalion Pipe Band gone. Did he ever say a single word against the Army? No. He loved those years. He talked of the Guards with fondness, always. It just ended badly and he got through it, got on with it, adapted, and lived the best life that he could.

We had to become expert on something we never expected to have to experience. We had to help him deal with it as best he could, and to be fair he dealt with it well. He had a good life considering the circumstances. He owned his own flat, drove his own car, briefly had a marriage and had lots of good friends.

Thanks to Glasgow University, seeing him not as a 'schizophrenic' but as 'an employee with schizophrenia', he held down the same job in the security department for twenty-seven years. More importantly to him, he was the University's official piper, playing at graduations and other events, and there is a portrait of him hanging at the foot of the stairs from the hall where most of those events took place.

For Donald piping became a life-defining passion. He competed at a high level. The judges, like his employers, recognised that he could sometimes be 'out of form in the head', as once when my sons Rory and Calum and I went to see him compete in a Piobaireachd Society competition. It was top-end stuff but Donald's mind was wandering and the judges smiled kindly when he stopped prematurely, said 'bugger it, I was away with the fairies there, Sir', saluted and left the stage.

The last time he played was at the University's memorial for its former rector, Charles Kennedy who, despite having been leader of a different party to my own, was a close friend. The whole political establishment of Scotland seemed to be there, First Minister Nicola Sturgeon included. Donald didn't look well. He was struggling for breath even before we started. I knew the signs all too well and I said to him 'listen, I can do this on my own'. 'No,' he said, 'I'll do it. I liked Charlie.'

We led the procession into the quadrangle. But a third of the way round he was fighting for breath and had to stop, and I finished alone. He never played again. To lose his work and then his piping to *physical* ill health, after doing so well for so long with his *mental* ill health, was cruel. But he never complained. He got a set of electronic pipes – in fact being Donald he got himself more than one – which can be played without lung power. Fine for him in that he could continue to keep his piping fingers active. Less good for the rest of us as he really loved to talk; it meant he could play and phone us at the same time, something he had never mastered with the 'real' pipes!

When he became ill, I read up as much as I could on the illness, and I recall being hit with a real chill by a research paper which said that on average schizophrenics on powerful anti-psychotic drugs can expect to live twenty years less than the rest of us. Donald was sixty-two when he died. My Dad was eighty-two. Bang on. Don't get me wrong. Medication can help restore someone to the person they are supposed to be, unclouded by the illness. Medication helped give Donald long periods free of the voices in his head and the hallucinations that could otherwise reduce him to a sometimes terrified and other times aggressive human being. So the drugs worked. To an extent. But decades on such strong medication take their toll. When it came to fighting 'normal' illnesses like colds, flu and chest infections, the gaps between them got shorter and the quantity of 'normal' drugs required to treat them got larger. Added to which, when his main medication for the schizophrenia was altered to deal with physical illnesses and weight gain it seemed to send him haywire mentally. But which other illnesses can you think of where we would tolerate the medication taking twenty years off your life? We are a million miles away from the parity between physical and mental health promised in the NHS Constitution.

It is a source of real sadness to me that our last conversations were with the psychotic Donald, not the loving, giving, funny Donald who had brought so much to our lives by making so much of his own. At his funeral, there were many who had no idea his illness had been so severe. Only those who had cared for him in the final days knew the sick Donald, throwing himself around, refusing medication, tearing out his oxygen tubes, snarling and shouting at everyone. Orchid Ward was a new addition on his NHS map. But when Liz and I went from seeing his body at the bereavement centre to collect his belongings from the ward, the nurses sought us out, not just to offer their condolences, but to tell us how much they had liked him. 'Oh, you could tell he was a character,' said one. 'I know I shouldn't laugh but he was funny,' said another. They talked about Donald's listening to his piping CDs in there – loudly – and other patients saying they would never hear the bagpipes again without the hairs standing up on their necks and thinking of him. They knew that beneath the crazy stuff that the voices and the visions made him do and say, he was a great guy. The fact *nurses* could see it even as they had to restrain him, at the end with three staff members having to be in his room round the clock, underlined that.

Till our mother died, I never talked about Donald's

illness in public mainly because she didn't want me to. Not out of the shame and stigma that many people sadly still feel about mental illness. She was incredibly proud of him. It was more that, not enjoying having one son in the media spotlight, she worried that if Donald's head was in any way above the parapet, it could have made him even more vulnerable.

Donald, on the other hand, was totally up for it. Like a lot of mentally ill people, when he was well he thought he ought to be famous. And when he was ill he thought he already was. In his prime, he saw Sean Connery as a suitable actor to play him in the movie of his life. More recently he had begun wondering if George Clooney could do a good Scottish accent.

He was competitive about his illness. 'Saw you on the telly again talking about your psychotic breakdown, Ali. You heard voices once and you're like Mister Mental Bloody Health. Why don't they come and talk to a real expert?'

He was certainly an expert on living a good life with severe mental illness. We were planning to make a film together – centred on him – on living with schizophrenia. He got the telly bug from the film we made about bagpipes. My daughter Grace, when a film student, had begun to record interviews with Donald. So he would sit and tell her about the time he was in a waiting room, and the wall-plugs were talking to the lights about him while he was surrounded by people who were all discussing terrible things they were about to do to him. Then he would laugh and say 'absolutely mad innit Grace? And look at me sitting here now. Normal or what?'

How times and families change. I don't criticise my parents for this, as times then were indeed different, and parents were perhaps more trusting of medics, but in that first crisis, once Dad had seen Donald and spoken to the military medical personnel in Netley, the next day he decided to head back home to work. I suspect he may have not been keen for my Mum to see Donald in the state he was in at that time, added to which, Liz was still at school. Mum and Dad, and later Liz when the term ended, went to visit him at weekends, staying with Dad's friends from his days as a Hampshire vet, Wilson and Eileen Atkinson.

Apart from a part-time job at a petrol station, I had no reason to go back to Leicester after that first visit, but more than that I hoped I could aid Donald's recovery just by being around. So I stayed. I must also confess to an immediate fascination, once it had been accepted that I could spend the daytime hanging around with Donald, with some of the other patients, and those looking after them – think *One Flew Over the Cuckoo's Nest* but with uniforms. The grounds were spacious and quite pretty in parts, the interior austere; Donald's room was certainly more cell-like than the usual NHS ward. Daytime was spent mainly in a large room with an assortment of worn-out comfy chairs where the patients sat, some in silence, others bantering loudly, or reliving Army times. 'You got no worries in the Army, Don,' said in a deep East Midlands accent by one of his fellow patients, became one of those phrases Donald would remember and repeat many times, usually to raise a laugh, in the years to come.

The whole Netley episode sparked my already burgeoning interest in matters of the mind. In addition to talking to the other patients, I enjoyed chatting to the psychiatrists and nurses. It's fair to say some were more caring than others. It was a hospital, yes, but it was also military, and this was in an era when soldiers had to buy their way out of the Armed Forces if they wanted to leave prematurely, and one of the nurses admitted to me they had to keep an eye out for men who might be faking illness as a way of getting out for free.

For the time I was there, I spent the days with Donald and the fascinating assortment of characters he now found himself with, and the evenings out drinking and trying to find someone, preferably female and good-looking, who would take me home for the night. Donald had a car, which unfortunately at the time was parked back in Leicester. Without telling my parents, I went home to get it and drove back south so at least I had somewhere to sleep if Plan A in the pubs and clubs came to nothing.

Drink was already a big part of my life. It had been for some time. I was still under the legal drinking age when I had my first medical warning. I had been getting such bad rashes aged sixteen or seventeen that I finally went to see the GP at the top of our road, Welland Vale Road, in Evington, Leicester. Our usual doctor was on holiday. The locum asked me if I had been drinking very much. 'A bit,' I said. 'How much?' she asked. I halved the real number, took off a few more, and told her. 'Mmm,' she said. 'That's a lot. You need to be very careful.'

Down in Netley, I was anything but careful. Day with Donald. Night with drink. On one of my successful Plan A nights, I remember waking up standing stark naked while peeing into a wastepaper basket in the corner of a strange bedroom I had no memory of entering. I dressed quietly, hoping not to disturb the sleeping woman who I think I had met on the dance floor of a nightclub and whose name I didn't even know. I made off into the night and the backseat of Donald's little car.

Donald was a great support after my own 'not as psychotic as mine, Ali' breakdown in the 1980s and we went on a road trip visiting friends and relatives around Britain. He was great company: real glue in both close and extended family, and a very loving and supportive brother. 'I want to kick that Michael Howard's teeth down his throat,' he said after a particularly unpleasant attack upon me by the former Tory leader. And when I say 'after', yes, I mean immediately after but also one week after, a month, a year and five, ten years after. He really didn't like people who said bad things about his family. And he loved saying the same things again and again. He had a book full of mantras. 'You got no worries in the Army, Al.'

Donald was very clever but not very well educated (the reverse of a lot of people I know). I have no idea when his mind first started to go wrong. I've often wondered, though, whether those times when he just couldn't seem to get himself out of bed, which my parents saw as signs of teenage rebellion, were the first indications of his approaching illness.

He had many doctors, nurses and psychiatrists over the years. One of them once said to me: 'Donald is my greatest success story. Keeps his job. Owns his own flat. Drives himself. Stays active. Has a passion for his music. Has more friends than any of us. Has a positive attitude almost all the time.'

That last bit was certainly true. If we had ever made that film about Donald we were going to call it *The Happy Schizophrenic*. 'It is what it is, Ali. I got given a bit of a crap deal, but you've got to make the best of it, know what I mean?' It helped that, unlike me, he did do God and his faith was certainly a comfort.

He loved people and he loved life. If there had been an extended family vote – we have thirty-one cousins – to elect its most popular member, he would have walked it. He worked almost all his life. He didn't like hospital for all the obvious reasons but also because he didn't like to be a burden on the NHS, which he felt had already given him more than most. He adored his nieces and nephews and was obsessed with the idea that he should have something to leave to them, even though several of them already earned more than he ever did. He was a total giver.

There is not a day of my life since that phone call to my Mum that I haven't thought about Donald and his illness. Why him, not me, or Graeme, or Liz? How very different our lives became and yet how close we remained. The guilt I felt at not always being there when he was in crisis. The guilt I felt when my phone rang and I knew it would be him to have the same chat as an hour ago and so I would simply pick up, quickly say 'call you back in a minute' and put the phone down. Even though I know that he thought his family did everything we could to help him, I will always feel there is more that I could have done.

Whenever I have explored my depression, which I have, with psychiatry, with science, with dream analysis, with all manner of deep dives into the mind, I have never fixed on the one thing that might explain it best. But I think it might be Donald and his illness.

Traumatic experiences, especially when young, can often be precursors to depression. Donald's diagnosis, and my reaction to it, was certainly a traumatic experience. I still have intense dreams about walking into that cell-like, grey, windowless room where he was being treated, seeing that cross on the wall, and Donald growling 'he knows, you know'.

Whenever he was subsequently taken ill – when, usually, after a period of good health he suddenly decided he didn't have to take his medication for a while – and we would pitch up at whichever hospital he had been taken to, I had a lesser version of those same feelings I remembered from Netley. Fear. And powerlessness. They are not things I like to have to deal with. When I am depressed, I feel powerless over my feelings, and that can scare me.

Though Liz only visited Netley once, she has a vivid memory of a hot summer's day, and sitting outside on the grass, playing cards. 'I was wearing a T-shirt with a picture on the front and Donald was transfixed by it. He knew who I was, but he was heavily drugged. I was only sixteen, and I told myself that maybe he was just a bit "down in the dumps". But I found the whole experience really shocking. It shook me to the core.' Liz went on to have eating issues not long after his diagnosis, and is convinced of the link.

I had another traumatic experience with Donald about twelve years before Netley. It was a classic sibling row in our garden in Keighley. He was winding me up, I grabbed something he was playing with and ran away towards the house, Donald in hot pursuit. Our front door was partly made of glass and as he chased me over the threshold I slammed the door as he put his hand through, cutting his wrist and arm badly on the glass. The subsequent wound, just millimetres from the main artery on his wrist, required dozens of stitches and left him with a scar for life. I have had a propensity to faint at the sight of blood – and, perhaps linked, a profoundly irrational revulsion to ketchup (look up saltomaphobia) – ever since.

I don't know. I just don't know if any of that is relevant. But I found myself reliving it in my head as I wrote about it. So perhaps it is. And maybe, again I don't know, maybe that was the reason I felt the need to stay in Netley and do my best to ensure he was, well, OK.

Liz was the last person to visit Donald, shortly before the respiratory collapse which led to his death. In those final days he had become unusually violent as the voices in his head became more and more unmanageable. After being admitted, he initially refused to take medication or even oxygen and was having to be restrained regularly. Once he had been stabilised somewhat, Liz took in some old family photograph albums and also some of his own recordings. And though he had forgotten a lot about himself and some of the people in the albums, and was back talking the same kind of paranoid nonsense we heard more than forty years ago in Netley, once she turned on the music, Donald's eyes lit up and his fingers started to play along with the tunes on the bed rail.

He lost his mind from time to time. Now, all too young, he had lost his life. But right to the end of it, he never lost the music in his soul. And though the Donald who died was the sick Donald, the workings of his mind divorced from people and events around him, in there somewhere was the real Donald. The real Donald left behind so much grief precisely because he inspired so much love, and gave so much love to so many, not least his little brother. The portrait at Glasgow University – which he would have loved – was paid for by his seven nieces and nephews out of the money he left to them. One of them, my sister's son Jamie Naish, wrote a song for Donald, which he played and sang, beautifully, at the funeral.

I've been in that place
Where the stars are blue
When it rains all day
Though you don't want it to

Nothing bright to see
No horizon to find
All alone in this world
A world that's borne of my mind

My mind has taken over
Over my life

The voices are so loud
Drowning out all other sounds
My mind's a beating drum,
Tells me evil's ways have won

The crowds, they laugh at me
Codes and words are all I see
Can't share a joke, a laugh, a smile
While the world is in denial

My mind has taken over
Over my life

So listen to me now
I'm a person, not a clown
This life is not a game
It's a fight I choose each day

So pick me up when I am down
Dare to turn my world around
Fight the demons here with me
Boy, I could use the company

My mind has taken over
But my life, it isn't over
Hello world, give me a shoulder
That I can cling to

That I can cling to
Let me cling to . . .

'My mind has taken over . . . but *my life*, it isn't over.' Donald's attitude to his illness is captured right there. His life was a struggle. But he really did live it, to the full, to the end, and I still miss him every day. I miss Graeme too, but with a sense of regret that he did not live the full life he could have done, given his real talents. Donald, by contrast, could look back on a life of which he made as much as he could, and though he knew the pain and misery of awful illness, he knew happiness and fulfilment too.

So now there are just the two of us: Liz and me. The youngest of the four of us, with three older brothers who occasionally teased her, Liz became an emotional centre of our family from a young age. She was always the one who showed most concern over, and the most care for, the rest of us. A teacher and accomplished pianist, and the mother of triplets, she has inherited our

Mum's role in being the one most on top of any news about extended family. It is no accident that our parents, and both our brothers, moved in later life to be near her home in Nottinghamshire, and she cared for all four with a dedication matched only by – and perhaps also driven by – the depth of her faith in God.

We were raised as Presbyterians, with weekly visits to church and Sunday school until my teenage rebellion put a stop to it, but our parents' faith was as much about a social life, and Mum's love of singing hymns, as it was about belief. It was as an adult that Liz developed a deeper faith. She doesn't push it down my throat, but I think she feels that if only I had the same relationship with God and Jesus that she does, my troubles would be eased, if not over. She might be right, and I know my atheism pains her. I have felt deeply spiritual at times, but it has never translated into the kind of faith she has. Despite our differences, we have always been close, and are especially close now, as we concentrate on crossing our next hurdle as siblings, of turning sixty-three safely. In my case, I'm approaching that hurdle all too soon.

2

LACHIE

Our summer holidays were very much family affairs, the six of us squeezing into Dad's car, the journey full of the usual games and squabbles, a stop for fish and chips in a place called Shap in Cumbria, then heading off to stay with an assortment of aunts, uncles and cousins in various parts of Scotland, before ending up in Tiree.

It is a small, treeless island, harsh in winter, but in summer Tiree boasts the longest spells of sunshine anywhere in the UK, and though now something of a surfers' paradise, back then it was possible to have its stunning white sand beaches all to ourselves. The long boat ride from Oban, free at last to run around after hours in the car, was one of the highlights, when Dad would get out the pipes and play them on deck as if to remind himself he was at last heading home.

We stayed either with Dad's younger brother Hector, who ran the family croft, Corrairigh, or his older sister Netta, who lived a hundred or so yards up the road with her husband, Alasdair Brown, and their three sons. Our Gaelic-speaking cousins, Margaret, Lachie and George

Campbell in Corrairigh, and Colin, Lachie and John-Neil Brown up the road at The Brae, had a very different childhood to ours – growing up as we did with English accents in a northern industrial town – but we got on pretty well and generally had a good time.

When I finally agreed to see a psychiatrist, not long after leaving Downing Street, he asked me if I could remember a feeling as a child that resonated with how I felt whenever I was depressed as an adult. The deepest memory I recalled came from one of these summer holidays. I was playing in a makeshift football match, jumpers as goalposts, five a side, at the local school. Unsurprisingly to anyone who knows me, I have always been somewhat obsessed with football, and with winning. My determination to do so on this occasion led to another boy – I think his first name was Ronnie – feeling I was both playing too well and too aggressively, a tendency to which I freely admit.

After I fouled him, he fouled me, and we ended up in a fight, which I lost. Badly. My excuse was that he was bigger and older than me but the pain of the humiliation was as great as the pain inflicted by the several decent punches he landed. I skulked away before the game was over, walked for a mile or so, then sat on a grassy rock about a mile from the family croft, before letting the tears pour out. What I remember most was the feeling of being absolutely on my own, and that I had to learn from and accept it. There had been nobody there to help me this time, and I had to be ready for whenever that situation, that feeling, might arise again.

So once the tears had stopped, I vowed I would tell nobody what had happened, laugh off my cuts and bruises as the result of an everyday football clash, and learn to look after myself better. It was probably a terrible mistake. It is one thing to learn to rely on yourself physically. But mentally and psychologically, one of the hardest things about depression is that feeling of utter isolation and helplessness.

I might like to think I can get through it alone, and for decades I did, or thought I did. But I can't. It has taken me years, and many depressive episodes fighting in solitude and in silence, to learn that. How much easier might I have found it if I had always been able to be as open as I am now, with family, with friends, with colleagues? How much might that openness have helped Graeme if he could have found it within himself to say to me, to any of us, to anyone at all, 'I'm struggling a bit here'?

How much better it is, when the dark cloud begins its descent, that I can say to Fiona, 'oh no, here we go again', rather than, as before, take it as a cue simply to turn my face against the world, lonely, desolate, disbelieving that anything or anyone could help me. How much luckier am I that among my friends there are a couple that I can always tell – 'having a really shit day' – and they will usually say or do something that helps.

Of all my cousins on Tiree, I was closest to Lachie Campbell, three years my junior, even if we had the odd scrap and argued a lot about who was the better piper. Lachie was the first of our generation of the family to achieve a fame of sorts. A film-maker, Bob McIntosh, was visiting Tiree to check out locations for a film about a boy and a seal. *Sula* was a fictitious Hebridean island, Tiree one of the real ones identified as a possible location for a film about a teenage boy's life there, and his relationship with the seal. He spotted Lachie, and something about his look, his walk, his determined features and then, when they talked, his voice and his accent, made him realise he had found the boy no casting director had been able to come up with for the lead role, Magnus MacDuff.

Lachie was an entertainer: he sang, played music and was an excellent mimic, especially of our grandparents, though he never quite mastered our Yorkshire accents. But he had no actual acting experience. Nonetheless, McIntosh took a punt on him and *Sula* was made in 1975, when Lachie was in his mid-teens, and was sufficiently successful for a sequel, *Return to Sula*, to be made three years later.

In such a small community, it meant he stood for something. Everyone knew everyone else, and everyone knew that Lachie had starred in a film. It was quite a thing, for him and for the island. It gave him a taste of stardom, not to mention the money to supplement the family earnings from the croft, and inspired a desire to be an actor, which he never quite achieved. His acting fame was short-lived, the child star whose career never made it to adulthood. Instead, after school, he went to

Agricultural College in Cupar, Fife to train as an agricultural engineer, then to Glasgow to serve his apprenticeship with Erskine Tractors.

He returned to Tiree, married Rosaleen in 1981, and they set up their family home in the cottage next to his parents. Crofter, fisherman, pier master, general man about the island: he was a big part of the community, not least in helping start the Tiree Feis in 1990, a festival to promote the language, culture and music of Tiree.

When we were young, and the Tiree Pipe Band was struggling for numbers, on holidays my Dad, Donald and I would help out. There is something very powerful about a good pipe band, the pipes properly tuned, players in harmony, drummers banging out the beat, and I know it meant a lot to my Dad and Uncle Hector that Donald and I turned out for them in this way. I recall vividly going by boat to play on the neighbouring island of Coll, the sea calm and flat on the outward journey, wild and stormy on the way back. Drink had been taken by all but the youngest of us. Never have I seen so many men being so violently ill over the side of a boat. Lachie was certainly in good mimicking form when we got back, and for days after reminded 'the men' how ridiculous they had looked and sounded as they threw up excessive quantities of whisky into the sea.

The long summers we spent on the island as children were among the happiest parts of our childhood and I envied Lachie's sense of belonging and commitment to the island. As numbers of inhabitants dwindled, the

Pipe Band fell into abeyance. Lachie made it his mission to help restore it.

So why, of my thirty-one cousins, am I singling out Lachie? The answer is that he is another reason I feel compelled to campaign for better mental health. Because at a time when I was busy as hell working for Tony Blair, early this century, exactly a month after we had seen in the Millennium with the Queen at the over-eventful launch of the Dome, came one of those calls you will never forget.

The phone rings. My Mum.

'Bad news, Ali.'

'What?'

'Lachie from Corrairigh has hung himself.'

What can you even say? It makes me so angry when someone takes their own life, and people who had never even met them say, 'didn't they think about the people left behind, how they would feel? Those poor children.' I would be surprised if Lachie thought of anything else but his poor children – Edward, Mairi Lyndsey and John. But this is something I know of: suicidal ideation. I have done it myself. I lie wide awake in bed, I can't sleep, feeling like death inside, dark stubborn pain eating into every cell of my body, my head both empty yet also somehow full of awful thoughts. Then what feels like a better thought pops in . . .

How peaceful, how beautiful does Fiona look? When she is asleep she can forget about me and about my moods. The minute she wakes my mood will define her day. And the next day. And the next. Because when you're depressed it feels this is the state you are going to be in forever. It doesn't matter that you have got through the same kind of thing before. It doesn't mean a thing because every time feels like the first time.

I sometimes compare it with childbirth. I find it very hard to see how a woman who has done it once would put herself through the same thing again. It is only because pain has no memory that she is able to. The pain of depression has no real memory.

Sitting here typing this, feeling OK, I cannot really describe what chronic depression feels like. I certainly cannot summon up the feelings. So when it comes on, the despair and desolation feel fresh and new, every time.

She would be so much happier if I was gone and she didn't have to deal with this shit, I tell myself. She would be sad I was dead, of course she would, and shocked if she were to find the body. She would scream, then cry, for a bit. She would steel herself to tell the kids, probably with her brother Gavin or her mother Audrey, or maybe Liz, at her side. That would be awful. But the funeral would be healing and then she would start to build a new and better life without me. The kids would rally round. They will be sad for a bit but it will be better for them too not to have to worry about what kind of mood dad is going to be in any more, whether he is going to be high as a kite thinking he can save the world, or lying on the sofa not wanting to see or speak to anyone. I mean, as a child I couldn't imagine being without my parents, but they're both gone now, and

I've survived, I've got over it. Fiona and the kids will get over it.

And then almost before you know it, you've got a pen and a piece of paper and you're writing the note, and it's like you are doing it for them, ending the pain inside for yourself, sure, but also for them. I once found a scribbled note on my bedside pad – 'AC death – short-term pain, long-term gain', like it was a tax hike or a staff sacking. Though I have no memory of how I felt when I wrote that, it doesn't take much to see how someone in that mindset might step from planning to deed.

By this point you're planning the funeral and deciding who you want to do the readings or the main eulogy. Tony Blair's the obvious choice I guess, but then I would also be hoping there would be a good turnout from Burnley FC past and present, and it might be nice to have one of my non-media, non-politics friends. Tim Kerr-Dineen from Cambridge University days perhaps, with such a different background to mine, my one really posh friend (apart from Tory MP Alan Clark, already gone), who always had that amazing bond with Donald because of their shared experiences of mental illness, and who made such an effort to come to his funeral. Syd Young or Geoff Lakeman from my early *Mirror* days, but then Syd would get overwhelmed by emotion, I know, and maybe Geoff should play his squeezebox instead, and entertain all our old journalist friends with his song 'Boys of the Byline Brigade'. Down it goes in the notebook. I'd definitely want Lachie's son John playing the pipes, with my cousin Susan's son Gavin Law, who was taught by Donald, and my friend and later-life piping tutor Finlay MacDonald from the National Piping Centre in Glasgow; and I want the Scottish folk band Skipinnish to play 'Forever Young' – Angus MacPhail, who wrote it, says I was the inspiration! – and 'Alive', as a message to people as they leave. 'Feel the wonder of the world, you are alive.'

I wonder if Lachie went through the same thought process, taking his life not just because he felt desolate, but because he felt it would be a release for Rosaleen and the children, a chance for them to live again, without the shadow of his drinking and his depression. I suspect he did.

When the last family member of my Dad's generation on the island, Auntie Mairi, died last year, she was laid to rest not far from where Lachie is buried. Once John and I had piped his grandmother's coffin to her grave, we went over to Lachie's. Overlooking Balinoe beach, it is one of the most beautiful burial spots anywhere on earth, and Lachie has the plot closest to the sea. John and I played on as other members of the family laid flowers. Mairi Lyndsey, eighteen when he ended his life, now a mother herself, the life she had spent without her dad now longer than the life she had with him, cried uncontrollably.

She and I talked for ages later. If we don't do God, as neither she nor I do, it is hard to make sense of the loss that we all experience in life, but which she, her mum and her brothers have experienced more deeply and more cruelly than most. The point, I said to Mairi Lyndsey, is that it is only because we have loved that we feel such pain, and the love merits the pain that follows its loss. We can still love people who are gone, and they can still influence how we feel and how we act. These are the things that make death at least understandable, if not bearable at the time. I said Lachie was with her, and he would be proud of the way she, Edward and John loved and looked out for their mum, and the way they had looked after and cared for Lachie's mum. He would have been proud of the way John and Edward were able to stand up in the church and sing a Gaelic lament, and of John's wonderful piping and his ridiculously smart kilt suit.

Auntie Mairi's funeral, by one of life's strange little coincidences, had fallen on the anniversary of Lachie's death on 31 January 2000. Auntie Mairi had felt Lachie's loss deeply. On one of my visits to her, she admitted she 'loved the pipes but hated the drinking that went with it', and when I left she gave me an envelope. 'I want you to have this, and read it, and keep it forever.' It was a printed copy of the eulogy read at Lachie's funeral by Jessie Gray.

Jessie's eulogy ended with these words. 'The circumstances which have led to us being here today are dreadful, tragic, sad, heart-breaking', but then she went on: 'About twenty minutes after being asked to speak here, I opened a book I had just bought, and on the first page there was a quotation from *Paradise Lost* by John Milton.

The mind is its own place, and in itself
Can make a Heaven of Hell, A Hell of Heav'n.

'Let us hope that Lachie's troubled mind has at last found peace and gentle rest.'

Mairi Lyndsey, Edward, John, Rosaleen, Uncle Hector and Auntie Mairi wouldn't have been human without asking all the questions people ask when someone we love ends their own life. What was he thinking? How did it get so bad? Could we have stopped it? Could we have done something differently? Was there something we missed? These questions are inevitable, but ultimately fruitless.

Lachie was loved. But sometimes the mind cannot see all the good in its midst, can only feel whatever pain there is to feel. I haven't done what Lachie did, nor actively tried it, but I've been very close, and I've known the feelings that take you there.

I told Mairi Lyndsey none of us would ever know what was going through Lachie's mind as he set up that rope on the beams beneath the red roof, but I knew that whenever I have been in those dark places, one of the main feelings I have had is that Fiona, Rory, Calum and Grace would be far better off without me. Sometimes when the pain of whatever feeling is tearing me up inside gets so strong, I think 'anything will be better than this'. My rational mind knows both those statements are nonsense. But the mind isn't always rational, and we cannot always control its thoughts, or the actions to which they lead us.

My point to Mairi Lyndsey was that for all the pain she has felt for the whole of this century, the love she showed for her grandmother and her dad at their grave-sides that day was one they felt just as deeply for her, and their love will be with her always. With every tear that fell, her love for them, and theirs for her, poured out.

That day felt like the end of an era, the last of that generation on the island going, its population now down to six hundred from the several thousands when my Dad was born, and most of those six hundred were there at the funeral.

But the end of one era also means the beginning of another. When Rosaleen and John drove me to Tiree's tiny airport overlooking Crossapol beach, we bumped into a young man from Glasgow named Scott Wood, who was waiting for the same flight as me. He came over to us and said he was 'Donald's replacement'.

For a few moments, I was confused. Then it clicked. One of Donald's sidelines had been as piping tutor to children on the island, by Skype and in person on regular visits, and when he died, I kept his best pipes, and donated his other sets – he was a bit of a hoarder – to the school. This was the school on whose football pitch I was beaten up over half a century ago. The school where Lachie was a pupil when he was spotted by a holidaying film-maker, and turned into a child star.

All death is hard, all grief is painful, but none greater than that caused by suicide. It lives with loved ones left behind for so much longer, precisely because we never stop asking those questions, for the truth is we can never fully know the answers. Had we done so, would we not have seen it coming, done something to stop it? All three of Lachie's children admit to his death having given them their own difficulties at times. They told me as much when I sent this chapter to them, to be sure they were fine with what I was saying. I was especially pleased by something that Edward said to me: 'It helps to read about it. It helps to understand. It helps to hear you say he wouldn't have wanted to hurt us.'

This strikes me as a feeling families affected by suicide need to have, and should hold onto, which is why the 'selfish' narrative is so harmful. Jessie Gray's eulogy to Lachie stayed in the inside pocket of one of my coats until, annoyingly, I left the coat on a train taking me to a Burnley game, and had to ask Mairi Lyndsey to send me a copy.

She included with it a poem that had been given to her and the family as part of a 'survivors of suicide pack' nineteen years ago. She says she reads it from time to time, to remind herself of what might have been going through his mind, and she recently sent it to a friend whose aunt had lost her son to suicide, just as my Auntie Mairi had. It ended like this:

I did not mean for you to grieve, now left alone
   to cry,
It wasn't my intention to leave you asking why.
As the burdens of life's worries ebb slowly from
   my heart,
It wasn't my intention to tear your soul apart.

I still occasionally watch *Sula* and *Return to Sula*, not merely to recall Lachie, his voice, his walk and his mannerisms, but also to remind myself how he lives on so clearly in his three children, children he loved, yet, in his pain, left behind with broken hearts that no amount of time will ever fully heal.

3

MY DEPRESSION SCALE

So Lachie hit ten on my mental health scale. It is a one to ten scale that I set for myself every morning as I wake. So much of the day ahead will depend on that first feeling, and the mark I give to my mood.

One is pure, unadulterated happiness. Ten is actively suicidal. I never hit, or even acknowledge, either of those, deliberately. One, for me at least, is unattainable. No matter how good I feel, and on many days I do, there is always something to make me restless or anxious. Sometimes it is the fear, born of experience, that the sensation of being close to pure, unadulterated happiness can be the precursor to crippling, howling depression. So, no matter how loved and lucky I may be – I am both – no matter how motivated I might be to face the day, two out of ten is as good as I allow it to get. Just as one is a no-go zone, so is ten. I don't like even to acknowledge that ten might arise, because in my rating system it is the number you reach when you decide not only that the pain inside is so unbearable that death would be preferable, but you also act upon it. Lachie hit ten. My highest ever has been nine.

So if one and ten are out of bounds, how does the rest of my scale work? Two feels great. I wake, having slept well; Fiona is alongside me and I feel blessed that she has stayed with me for four decades of considerable ups and downs; I have a day ahead that will keep me busy, motivated, doing something vaguely important I hope, putting what an old friend described as my 'demonic energy' to good use; I will also have time for exercise and music. Three and four are slightly down-scale variations on the same themes.

If any of the children are unhappy, that can definitely knock the rating upwards a mark or two. We are, after all, never happier than our least happy child, and all three of ours have given us moments of worry, small and very large. Tiredness and bad dreams can add a point to the rating. Politics can do it too. Brexit, climate change, Donald Trump, Boris Johnson in Downing Street, the state of today's Labour Party, all occasionally provoke an upward tick. Five is when I start to worry. Waking thoughts will be about things I have to do, but suddenly I don't feel so motivated to do them. I have to force myself to get out of bed. Shaving, brushing my teeth and getting dressed become not merely irritating chores, but tiring.

It is when I am in the middle of the scale that it most helps to have it. Five is the beginning of the danger zone, where the warning lights start to flash. Take a wrong turn, and a spiral towards six, seven, eight, nine can come all too easily. Seven is basically the signal to cancel meetings, stay indoors, avoid people, waste time, ruminate; and when that slips to eight and nine, to get into bed and sleep as much as possible because then at least you are not conscious of the feelings so much.

Five and six, then, are the key. Once they come on, it is vital to try to stop them from going higher. So I have my little tests. Shaving is vital. It is amazing how often depressed men have stubble. Shaving is one of the first things that goes for me. Brush teeth. Wear proper clothes. Try to work. Try to read. Try to eat. Try to do some exercise. Try to listen to or, even better, play some music. I mightn't succeed with all or even any of them, but if I do, it helps slow the slide.

There is a blind on the landing outside our bedroom. I force myself to open it. That mundane act has sometimes held me at five or even got me back to four. If I walk past the blind without opening it, it means I'm already at six. Seven is when others start to notice, especially Fiona. The stubble. The scruffy clothes, unchanged from yesterday. Not wanting to eat breakfast. Turning off the radio because the noise does my head in.

By seven, even the act of speaking is hard – not easy if the day ahead includes talks or interviews. At seven, I can still do them, hoping I get a little lift out of a change in scenery. So out I go, to go through the motions, and at the end I will feel both dissatisfied at my own performance and exhausted by the effort required. With eight, I will try to clear out as much of the day's diary as I can, certainly no social engagements, only professional ones that really cannot be called off. At nine, even they go, because now bed is the only place to be.

Some have suggested that I have my scale the wrong way round and that one should be suicidal and ten deliriously happy. I see their point. But I want to have suicide as the peak. Because suicide is the ultimate in mental illness, when the pain going on in the mind is so strong that death becomes preferable to life.

Self-harm is a downscaled version of the same thing. The self-harm of a young girl cutting her arm repeatedly with a razor is only the most obvious form of it. Alcohol and drug abuse are another form of self-harm. Any addiction is self-harm. I have known addiction, I have known self-harm, and not long after I left Downing Street in 2005, amid one of the worst and most prolonged bouts of depression of my life, I inflicted on myself one of my worst experiences of physical self-harm.

Partly I think I was going through decompression. I had for over a decade operated under a level of pressure, which, my GP Tom Bostock once told me, most people would not tolerate for a day or a week, let alone a year or a decade. I had gone from having clear and complete professional purpose to a diary of empty days stretching out before me, and the panicky feeling I had to start all over again.

I might have left Downing Street, but the key people in politics, especially Tony Blair and Gordon Brown, would not allow me to move on. This was not helped by the large part of me that didn't want to, feeling as I did that I had left as much due to pressure from Fiona as from deciding that I really had hit the end of the road. And all the while the issue of Iraq was continuing to haunt the government, ensuring my name stayed pretty central to a debate over which I now had much less influence or control.

It was not a happy time for me or for the family. I remember Labour minister David Blunkett coming for dinner one evening and Grace talking to him as she played with his guide dog Sadie and I took a call from Tony – he was still calling me most days, sometimes several times – in the hallway. David and Grace's conversation vividly brought home to me how I must be coming over, and just how vacuous that old cliché – 'I am leaving to spend more time with the family' – must sound.

'Is it nice having your dad home more?' asked David.

'Mmm,' said Grace, unconvincingly, as she stroked the dog.

'What does he do with his time now?'

'Well, when I go to school in the morning, he sits where you are on the sofa having a cup of coffee. And when I come back at the end of the day he is lying on the sofa fast asleep.'

It was unsustainable. Something had to give. So something did and I exploded. Not then, not with David and Grace chatting away, but a few days later. The depressions would not go. The pain would not subside. Fiona, though we were still going through a period of intense recrimination – she blamed me for bringing so much pressure into the family, I blamed her for forcing me out of the role I felt I was made for – was really trying her best and suggested we go for a walk to talk things over. Again.

The day before we had had a massive argument when she had launched a full-on assault on Labour education policy, saying our departure from Downing Street now meant she should be free to say what she wanted. And now she was badgering me to go with her to an event in Parliament where she, former Labour leader and long-time close family friend Neil Kinnock and others would continue the assault, and I knew the media would be looking at me for my reaction.

As we walked through one of the woods near Kenwood House, I felt the pain inside combining with rage about it not subsiding, and the seeming inability of the two of us to get on, and I began to punch myself repeatedly in the face. Hard. Bruisingly hard. Harder than the boy Ronnie had hit me fifty-odd years ago. My jaw and my right eye socket already felt numb. Fiona put her hands to her mouth, looking terrified, as I carried on punching. She wasn't terrified that I was going to hit her – I never would – but she was scared for me. I was losing my sanity. I was self-harming, hoping the pain of those punches on the outside could somehow drive out the pain on the inside. She said later she thought it was just me feeling so wretched inside. But I think it was more that I felt as if I would never see the back of my depression because the circumstances that worsened it kept crowding in on me.

Does the scale help? I find it does. Ruling out one and ten helps, but I have definitely been at nine. In Australia recently, where I was announced as a global ambassador for Australians for Mental Health, a new advocacy group, a road transport official talked to me about the official suicide statistics. He said the real figures were totally underestimated 'because so many road traffic deaths which are classed as accidents are actually almost certainly suicides'. That really resonated with me. It is one of the ideations I have regularly had come into my mind when on a seven, eight or nine.

When the Hutton Inquiry into the death of government weapons inspector David Kelly was underway, I got a fax on holiday in France saying Lord Hutton wanted to see my private diaries. (Maybe Fiona has a point. So many of our family holidays have been overtaken by my work from the time Tony and his family turned up to persuade me to join him, to Robin Cook, the then Foreign Secretary's affair being exposed, to the Omagh bombing, or the weeks spent working on drafts for the upcoming post-holiday Party Conference speech.) Getting that fax, however, was a horrible shock that made me feel – here we go again – scared and powerless. Scared because God knows what he would make of the things I said to myself late at night in the privacy of my own diary. One wrong word, and it could be the end not just of me, but the government. No wonder Tony sounded so panicked when I told him, so desperate for me to challenge the request. And powerless because I alone was being asked to do this, and I knew I couldn't say no. As I said to him: 'You have asked a judge to conduct an inquiry. You have said you and your staff will cooperate. He has asked for my diary as part of that cooperation. On what basis do I say no?' He called incessantly over the next few days, asking if I had transcribed them yet, what was the worst thing in there, 'you and your bloody diary' . . .

TB: Is there much swearing?
AC: Yes.
TB: What is the worst?
AC: Cunt, probably.
TB: You or me saying it?
AC: Both.
TB: Oh fuck, Alastair.

Fiona was trying to be supportive but I could tell she was furious with me that this was what our life on 'holiday' had become, and her total opposition to the Iraq war was compounding the fury. The Kinnock family was staying nearby, and I sought solace with them. Neil shared my rage but urged me to stay calm; his daughter Rachel is one of my favourite people in the world, always able to see the funny side of life, but even she could not really keep my spirits up. Their saying 'I'm sure it will be OK' felt more like hope than judgement.

There was an additional complication – the diaries were in London and I was in France. We had to get Fiona's mum, Audrey, to find them in the house, hand them to a Number 10 clerk who flew with them to

Marseille, was met off the plane by the head guy from the British Consulate, who handed them over to me so I could meet up with my newly appointed lawyer, Jonathan Sumption, to whom I would have to read every word for the period in question, so he could decide what would be deemed relevant to the inquiry. Then we had to arrange for my PA Alison Blackshaw to come out to help transcribe them. It was also in the middle of one of the worst heatwaves France had ever endured.

On the drive to the airport, and on the drive back – the diaries sitting on the passenger seat, me scared to open them, Fiona and Tony repeatedly calling to ask if I had, Tony wanting to know what they said, Fiona suggesting I just 'throw them in the swimming pool and sod the lot of them' – I came as close as I have ever done to becoming one of those road traffic accident stats that is actually a suicide. It was a fight to resist the desire just to pull off the road and drive at top speed into a tree or a truck coming the other way.

Eventually I pulled into an *aire* (a halfway house between a lay-by and a service station), parked in the shade of a huge willow tree and sat there trying to calm myself. I compared how I was feeling to how I felt at my worst, psychotic meltdown in 1986. That was a nine. How bad is this? Six, maybe seven. Come on. You can get through it.

Then my phone rang. It was my deputy, Godric Smith, just calling for a chat. He was unaware I had been asked for my diaries. He was unaware I had been advised to get my own independent legal advice. He exploded, on my behalf, at the unfairness. 'Why only you? Why doesn't he ask if [Andrew] Gilligan or [Greg] Dyke [two of the key BBC figures involved in the dispute with the government] keep a diary? Why only you?'

Then he exploded at the fact that he, who was also being called to the Inquiry, had been given no advice from the Cabinet Office, let alone his own expensive 'brain the size of a planet' lawyer like Sumption. Normally so mild-mannered – he had once been described as 'Chris Tavaré to [my] Ian Botham' (apologies to non-cricket fans) – his explosion was so huge it became comic, and helped my suicidal feelings pass.

I think of Godric every time I pass that *aire*. I can smile at it now. It also means that, in addition to being my former deputy, he is a good friend, and on my list of the people I know can sometimes, just by chatting, help to lift me up the scale. Because he did it once before. Most on that same list have an instinct for when I am not quite right. Often, it is the voice that is the giveaway. My voice literally weakens as I tumble down the scale. I sound quieter, hoarser, a bit reedy. It is a particular drawback when so much of my work involves speaking. I have a voice scale all of its own. When my voice starts to go into five, six or seven, I know my mind is going and I am already in the danger zone. (It's a good job, then, that here at least we are dealing in the written word, not the spoken word.) But for now, I want to try to answer the question, for those who have not known depression . . . what is it like?

4

WHAT IT FEELS LIKE

I've had times in my life when I have been sad, but not depressed; and times when depression has not been the same as an acute form of sadness. They can be very different things, and that's what people who don't have direct experience of depression find very difficult to understand. They might imagine (and this is something that has been suggested to me many times) that you can change the way that you feel – but when you're depressed you can't. That's when it gets really hard. It's like thinking you can stop the rain from falling, or the sun from shining.

So, what is it like? How do you begin to describe something like depression? All I can do here is describe my own. I have heard many other people describe theirs, and there will certainly be points of resonance. Yet, just as all minds are unique, I suspect that all depressions are too. So I can try to give you a sense of mine, with the unhelpful caveat that while there are certain similarities that draw my depressive bouts together, there are differences too.

It usually – though not always – starts as I wake. I might have been feeling myself dip down the scale the night before. I might have slept badly, or had unusually troubling dreams. As I wake, my head feels a little heavier than usual, and I have a desire to go back to sleep, but can't. I lie on my back, stare at the ceiling, and to my left, about six to eight feet away, I have a sense of a dark grey cloud, oval, about five times the size of a rugby ball, which fills me with dread. It has a colour, a texture and it has a feel, a kind of really unpleasant sort of jelly feel. I might talk to it: 'please, no, go away. Just fuck off.'

I close my eyes and in my mind's eye there is now a smile on the oval cloud, and it is moving in, slowly at first, then a little quicker, and I am trying to push it away, but I can't. Its smile is growing because the cloud knows I am about to give up the struggle and let it in. Reluctantly, I say 'come on then, let's get it over with', and then it is inside me, and it feels like a heavy liquid is being poured through my veins, and my body starts to join my mind in feeling heavy. The cloud has evaporated, but its smile is still there, and it is saying, 'Gotcha . . . again . . . you thought you were rid of me . . . no chance . . . I'm back, and this time I'm never going away again.'

In the old days, I would live with that feeling, get up, carry on, pretend I was fine, drink to drown the depression, work to chase it away. Now I tell Fiona straight away, 'I think I'm going down again.' She always asks, though she knows what my answer will be, 'what triggered it?' and I say 'I don't know.'

The strangest thing is feeling that you are empty inside, that you have been hollowed out, your real self has been evacuated from your body, and yet you're full too; full of something that has replaced it, this darkness, the cloud turned to heavy metal as it pours slowly around your insides. I see it as a brown-red sludge, slow but unstoppable, like the lava from a volcano. The dynamo I normally feel 24/7 whirring inside me, ready for action, energy waiting to be used, is switched off. Literally, you feel like there is a power cut, a switch has gone off and you don't know why, and you don't know who did it, but you know you are going to be scratching around your emotional bank to find a few candles to light to replace the bright lights that have suddenly gone. Energy gone. Power gone. Desire gone. Motivation gone. The ability to feel anything other than the numbing pain the cloud has brought about – gone. Everything gone, gone, all gone.

Even getting out of bed becomes a fierce struggle, the thought of doing it making you more tired, the heavy liquid feeling heavier inside. If I manage to move, I will then sit on the side of the bed for a while and engage in the next struggle – getting to the bathroom. Shaving has become hugely important to me when the cloud first lands. I try to force myself to do it. If I don't, I am in real trouble. Back to bed, fuck it, give up, let's not even try.

It is not purely psychological, for there is an almost physical feeling of pain, but nowhere you can point to and say 'it hurts there'. It hurts everywhere, uniformly, outside and, especially, inside. My voice weakens, and I have a mild but unpleasant metallic taste in my mouth. As to what I am feeling emotionally, yes, I am sad, but it is much worse than that. It is despair. Hopelessness. Hopelessness in both meanings of the word . . . I feel devoid of hope that my life will ever be good, and I feel pathetic, worthless, useless, that I have so much going for me and yet, yet again, this fucking cloud has come in, taken me over, beaten me.

Let's say I make it downstairs, or even out into the world, and get to a meeting. Whatever is going on around me, things that I would normally be interested in, I'm not. There is an existential feeling – 'I just don't want to be here'. I don't want to be with these people, right here, right now. And I just don't want to be here. Full stop. Now the depression is in full control, physically and mentally I have lost all power, and lost all will. I can literally see no point, in the moment or in the future. I can touch a pen, and know my senses are working. I can see someone is smiling at me, and force myself to smile back, but I know that I'm running on empty, and the forced smile makes me emptier still.

Dead and alive at the same time . . . I keep coming back to that as the best description. That is when, these days at least, I will vacate, say to Fiona that I just need a bit of time for this to pass, disappear. Out to the car, drive aimlessly, out on the Heath, walk aimlessly, anywhere I can be alone, and not have to speak. Here is where it is hard for partners. I want Fiona to be nearby, but I don't want her in my face. It is hard for me, and hard for her. But the openness we have found in recent years, me telling her when the cloud is coming, her understanding it is not her fault, this has really helped both of us.

As to how long it lasts, and how it leaves, again that varies. I would say four days is around average. Sometimes it's shorter, sometimes a lot longer. Sometimes I can feel like it's going, but then it doesn't. Sometimes its departure can be slow, a diminishing of the pain and the lethargy over a few days. Other times – this applies to the suicidal episode I described in the Preface – it can pass almost as quickly as it came. Just as I can never isolate the trigger that causes it, so I can never confidently identify the reasons why it goes. The heaviness starts to lift. Motivation starts to return. Energy starts to flow back. Sleep can help. Exercise can help. Music can help. Above all, getting on well in my key relationships helps, though I never quite work out whether the depression is lifting because I am getting on better with Fiona and the kids, or we are getting on better because the depression has lifted. Whichever, it is a sign that things are on the up again.

5

HITTING ROCK BOTTOM

It is the spring of 1986 and I am at the Labour Party's Scottish conference in Perth, to conduct an interview with their leader, Neil Kinnock, for a profile I am supposed to be writing for the soon-to-be-launched *Today* newspaper. The interview never happened because I became separated from him and his entourage, but now, thanks to his press secretary Patricia Hewitt, I am back with them and she is going to find some time for us to talk. But first he is speaking at a dinner in a council building in Hamilton, Fife.

I am standing in the foyer, enveloped in a kaleidoscope of sound. Some of those sounds – the voices of people talking as they file into dinner, bagpipes leading Neil to the top table – are real. But many are not. There are different pipe tunes playing discordantly inside my head; there are brass bands too; Abba and Elvis drift in and out; there are people shouting at me; me shouting back; people shouting at each other; and I am standing there thinking 'oh no, this is it, this is what happened to Donald'.

The fear that I too have schizophrenia sends my panic into a spiral. I ask a man with a badge – a council worker, I assume – if there is a telephone I can use. This was before near universal mobile telephony. But I know I must call home. He leads me up a staircase – I can feel his concern, it is fuelling my paranoia – and into the office of the chief executive. He points to a yellow phone on the large, leather-topped desk in the far corner, and leaves me there.

I ring Fiona. No reply. Weird – she said she was staying in, but that was before the massive row we had last night when I called home drunk to say I would not be back till late, and we both slammed the phone down on each other.

I had carried on drinking till closing time, then checked into that big hotel by Victoria station, emptied the mini-bar, woke up with my jacket and shirt covered in my own vomit, realised I had an 8 a.m. flight to Glasgow with Neil Kinnock and team, left the hotel without checking out, jumped in a cab to Heathrow, bought a new suit, blue shirt and red tie, dumped the vomit-stained ones in a bin in the gents, cleaned myself up and dressed in front of startled-looking fellow visitors to the bathroom, just made the flight, grabbed half an hour's sleep on the plane and hired a car at Glasgow airport to be able to follow Neil through the day. Then, dumping the car at Rosyth Naval Dockyard, realising Neil had left for Perth, I found another cab; I catch up with him, just catch the end of his speech, jump in a car with Patricia Hewitt to follow Neil and his wife Glenys to Falkirk Labour club – where I had my last drink – then to Hamilton. The madness is breaking, the voices are cacophonous, I keep calling home, and there is no reply; where the fuck is she, has she left me, was last night the final straw?

I phone my parents. No reply. My siblings. No reply. The office. No reply. I call half a dozen close friends whose numbers are in my head. No reply. No reply. No reply. No reply. No reply. No reply. Where the fuck have they all gone? Why is nobody home?

It is only later I learn that every time I dialled the first zero of every number I was trying, I was going through to an unmanned weekend switchboard. The thought – 'dial 9 for an outside line' – tends not to enter the psychotic mind, and even if the man with the badge had told me to do so, the message never got through the other noises in my head.

I walk back down the stairs, slowly, and return to the foyer. Again, the real noises are mixing with the imaginary ones but I can no longer tell which are which. A man in a kilt walks by, carrying bagpipes. He was probably one of the pipers who led Neil to the top table. I am sure – this is me in 2019 speaking now – he was real. I say to him – back in 1986 – 'Is this happening to me because of Donald?'

'Who's Donald?' he asks.

In the circumstances perhaps this was not an unreasonable response to a wild-eyed stranger asking an odd question. But 'who's Donald?' triggers all manner of fresh paranoid thoughts in me, up to and including the thought that Donald has been taken away and killed. 'Who's Donald?' He means 'Donald is no more.'

'Is Donald dead?' I ask.

'What the hell are you talking about?' I imagine he thought I was drunk, or on drugs. He walked on.

With Donald – possibly – dead, I fear I am now being tested for my own survival, and if I fail the test, I too will be killed. As part of the fight, I need to strip down to the bare essentials. Just me with my wits about me, nothing else required.

I empty my pockets and throw the contents on the floor. The fight for survival will be cashless. My wallet and money go. It will be borderless. I throw my passport in too. I have a shoulder bag with a few books, my diary, notebooks, a tape recorder, a washbag. I empty the items out one by one until I have a little circular pile developing. The noises are becoming deafening.

We all need luck, and a huge stroke of luck is about to strike.

It comes in the form of two men I see hovering out of the corner of my left eye, standing by the door through which the man in the kilt headed back towards the noise – the real noise – of the dinner about to be addressed by Neil Kinnock. They are both tall, very smartly dressed. They walk slowly towards me. I stand still. I stop emptying my bag. I throw it on the pile.

Tall Man One, grey suit, sharp white shirt and dark blue tie, dark Brylcreemed hair, speaks first.

'Are you OK?'

I look into his eyes, which do not for one moment veer from mine, and after a few seconds, I reply, softly, weakly: 'I don't think I am.'

Tall Man One nods, leaves the thought hanging, says nothing, keeps holding my gaze as I hold his. He has warm, compassionate, grey eyes.

A few more seconds pass, then Tall Man Two, dark suit, light blue shirt and dark tie, short, sandy hair, speaks.

'Do you think you should come with us?' he says.

I nod. 'I think I should.'

They could have been the Moonies for all I knew, but the next thing I know I am in a police car, then in a cell.

Later Patricia Hewitt has noticed I have gone missing, learns what has happened, calls in to tell the police I am who I say I am, and Patricia, who knows all about mental illness, having lost a sister in Australia to suicide, tells them she has been worried about me for some time and thinks I may need medical help.

By now I am in full paranoid flow. The police track down a journalist friend, Brian Steel, who lives nearby and comes to accompany me to hospital. I am assuming he is part of the plot against me, or else how did the police know where he was, know he is a friend, manage to find him late at night? The next day Fiona and her dad – by a remarkable coincidence, the hospital is in Paisley where he was born – fly up from London and arrive at my bedside. In my floods of tears, which erupt as they walk through the door, the road to recovery truly begins.

So what was the stroke of luck regarding those two plain-clothes police officers that I reflect on so often, not least when I walk past men and women living on the streets, lost to alcoholism and other forms of mental illness? It was not so much what happened, as what might have done.

What if – anyone who knew me as a young man would know this was not impossible when drink was taken – what if instead of admitting, for the first time, yes, I think I am struggling, when the first officer asked if I was OK, I had felt threatened, lashed out and head-butted him as his eyes locked on mine? Assaulting a police officer – we all know where that ends, and no amount of 'psychiatric reports ordered by the court' is going to stop it ending there.

'You had a good well-paid job, Mr Campbell, a good education, a loving partner, opportunities denied to people much less fortunate than you. These police officers were trying to help you and you threw that back in their face, violently. There can be no excuses for your behaviour. I sentence you to six months in jail. Take him down.' And then what? Back to journalism? Not so easy. Politics? No chance. Your life has changed mate, and it is never changing back. Every form you ever fill, when you get to that 'criminal record' bit . . . you're fucked.

I doubt those two policemen have given our encounter a moment's thought since. For them, it was just another incident on the mental health front line to deal with as they were looking after a visiting VIP. But

I think of them often. I feel they may have saved my life.

Stroke of luck Number Two came a few days later, in a phone call from my former boss, Richard Stott. I've been in Ross Hall Hospital a few days now and I'm sedated, sad, anxious. A very nice psychiatrist called Dr Ernest Bennie has begun to coax me to the view that the breakdown might have been influenced by a combination of overwork and alcohol abuse. The paranoia is still there, and whenever I watch TV or read the papers, I find myself doing complicated word and number games – very *A Beautiful Mind* – and trying to crack codes which I think will give me the keys to the door out, and freedom again. There are, in retrospect, some moments of pure comedy.

A friend and colleague from the *Daily Star*, Chris Boffey, was one of the people Fiona contacted when she got the call to say I had been arrested. So the nurse wheeled in the phone, and there was Chris on the end of the line. We chatted away, about football, my Burnley, his Manchester United, gossip, colleagues, and I asked if there was anything decent on the telly tonight.

'Taggart,' he said.

'Taggart,' I replied. 'What the hell is Taggart?'

'You know Taggart for God's sake. Everyone knows Taggart.'

'I don't.'

'It's about a Scottish detective. The one with a smile carved out of granite.'

Ping! New code alert!

'Thanks Chris,' I say, conspiratorially, and gently put the phone down. I have a new plan.

I could not contain my excitement as morning turned to afternoon, afternoon to evening, until finally it was time for Taggart. I studied Taggart's face. And there it was, halfway through the programme, the smile carved out of granite. I saw it so clearly. The new key to my freedom!

I went to the bathroom. I looked in the mirror, and practised and practised until I had perfected the Taggart look. I went back to bed, pressed the button to call in the nurse, and sat up straight as she entered, Taggart granite smile across my face, teeth touching on the right, left side of the lip rising slightly, eyes a mix of warmth and cold, hard menace.

'Yes?' asked the nurse.

I pointed to my mouth, to the smile, to the code being cracked, and waited for her to say 'well done, Alastair, you've worked it out. You can go.'

But she didn't. She said 'you just sit tight now, my love, I'll go and get the doctor.'

And they promptly upped the dose of whatever it was I was on.

I can laugh at it all now, but it's scary that your mind can take the turn that mine had done, to believe my future health and happiness depended on being able to impersonate the smile of a TV detective, or crack anagram codes based on the torrent of football teams and scores coming out of Des Lynam's mouth as he read off the BBC *Grandstand* teleprinter.

Bizarrely, many years later, the playwright Jimmy McGovern asked me to play myself in a TV drama, *The Accused*, in which a young man with psychosis was convinced whenever he saw me on TV that I was talking directly to him. It sounded fun, and interesting, and I had to go to Manchester for the filming, where I talked to McGovern over lunch in the location catering bus.

'I guess you asked me because someone told you about me and Des Lynam and Taggart?'

He looked at me like I was mad. He had no idea I had had psychosis. It was a total coincidence. He just thought I had the kind of profile for someone who might get inside someone's head when they were cracking up.

6

JOURNALISM

I can't really remember why I became a journalist. I had left university with no clear idea of what I wanted to do with myself, and drifted for a while, not unlike Graeme, with a part-time job here, there, always on the move. By then I knew I could always make enough money to live on busking with my bagpipes, which I did, in several parts of the world. I had always written a lot as a child – poems, songs, stories, diaries – and although I had never got into student journalism, I fancied myself as a sportswriter, and so began to hang around press boxes after football matches and cricket matches and try to get in with the big-shot journalists.

John Thicknesse, cricket writer on the *Evening Standard*, was a real help and got me a trial at a sports agency, Hayter's. Colin Hart of the *Sun* was another who gave me the time of day, and a bit of encouragement. But somewhere on the way, I must have become aware of the *Mirror Group*'s training scheme, applied for it, and was accepted. It was life-changing in two ways. It set me on course for my first career. Also, one of the other young trainees taken on at exactly the same time was a pretty Londoner, Fiona Millar. I knew as soon as I saw her that something was going to happen between us. And it did.

After some basic training in law, shorthand and how to write stories, we were sent to the *Tavistock Times*, and Fiona and I got a flat together. We spent a year there, then a year at what we called 'the Truro bureau' of the Plymouth-based *Sunday Independent*, living in Falmouth. By then we were so identified as a couple there was no question of our being sent to different papers in the *Mirror*'s West Country stable.

I felt like a round peg in a round hole as a journalist. It was an excuse to go up to anyone, and ask anything. It was an excuse too to walk into any pub you fancied, and imagine there was a story lurking in there somewhere, and often there was.

And then, my first big break, which was born, as were so many Fleet Street breaks, out of misunderstanding and exaggeration. It came courtesy of Richard Stott, at the time assistant editor at the *Daily Mirror*, after he – wrongly – heard I had hit *Mirror Group* panjandrum Bob Edwards when he made a pass at Fiona at a talk to the trainees in Plymouth. The truth was more prosaic: it was another of those drinking stories that got out of control. Bob Edwards was a friend of her dad and so asked to go out for dinner with us along with the head of the training scheme, Colin Harrow, after his talk. I drank too much, we had a row about a story he had run on page eight of the *Sunday*

Mirror that weekend saying the Falklands War was about to end, and I tapped him on the face (I thought playfully enough), suggesting if he had believed it, it should have been the front page lead. I was given a written warning the next morning, but by the time the bush telegraph reached *Mirror* HQ, I was the young buck who had laid out Bob Edwards for trying to steal his girlfriend. This was the kind of story journalists preferred.

When Fiona later went for an interview at the *Mirror* with the then women's editor Anne Robinson – yes, that one – I was waiting for her in the *Mirror* pub, the White Hart, otherwise known as the 'Stab' as in 'stab in the back'.

Suddenly, the door swung open loudly and in walked two men, both laughing. 'Where's the kid who thumped Bob Edwards?' one of them shouted out.

They spotted me drinking alone in the corner.

'Is it you?' asked a man I later learned to be John Penrose, aka Mr Anne Robinson.

'Well,' I stuttered, 'erm . . .'

'Good lad,' said the second man, who introduced himself as Richard Stott, 'best thing you've ever done. How do you fancy six weeks of shifts at the *Mirror* when you're done with your training?'

As I say, quite a break, and all for a drunken incident that never really happened. But who was I to argue? I thus became just the second *Mirror* trainee to go straight from the training scheme into the *Daily Mirror* newsroom, eventually being appointed full-time to the staff.

The first to make that journey had been John Merritt, my best friend in journalism then and for the rest of his life, and one of the finest reporters of our generation. Richard had risen to be *Mirror* editor by the time John and I were headhunted by *Today*, a new paper being launched by Eddy Shah, and offered bigger jobs with more money. Richard, who felt we were *Mirror* through and through, professionally and politically, was appalled we were even thinking of it. Eventually he persuaded John to stay. But I went.

It was, as Richard warned me it would be, a terrible mistake. Becoming the youngest news editor in Fleet Street was good for the ego of a twenty-eight-year-old, but I was not remotely ready for all that it entailed. I had been flattered into taking a job I should never have accepted. It was not the only reason for my breakdown, but the extra stress, leading to even heavier drinking, a worsening time at home and constantly feeling out of my depth but refusing to admit that to anyone, even myself, must all have been factors.

When I cleared my desk at the back of the newsroom to leave on my final day at the *Mirror*, Richard was watching me from the back bench where he was editing that night's paper. I can see him now: feet on desk, tie loose at the collar. He is looking straight at me, but without the cheeky, cheery smile that was never far from his face. In its place was a look that said 'never darken my door again'.

So when the phone was wheeled in to my hospital bedside again, and I picked it up to find Richard on the other end of the line, it was a shock.

'I hear you've gone mad,' he said.

'Well, I'm not well, for sure.'

'OK, well, I won't say I told you so . . .'

'You just did.'

'Ha! Yes, I guess so. But anyway, here is what you're going to do. And this time, old man' – he called everyone old man, whatever their age – 'you just *listen* to me. You stay where you are till the doctors say you are fit to leave. You go home and rest and recuperate. You then go back to that stupid newspaper where they can't even print photos without the ink running, and where I told you it would end in tears for you, but we won't dwell on that, and you work out your terms of departure. Then when you are a hundred per cent fit, you come back here, and we start all over again.'

Even as he spoke, I felt an enormous weight rising from my shoulders. I had been lying in that bed, manically cracking codes, manically writing notes to all and sundry – most, thankfully, never sent – obsessing I was trapped inside some Thatcherite re-education camp.

But once my mania calmed, one of the worst feelings was that my career was over. Word had spread that something had happened to young, high-flying, arrogant, know-it-all, cocky Campbell. The people I used to drink with were now standing at the bars where we drank – the Stab, the Poppinjay, the Cheshire Cheese, the Old Bell, the Press Club – swapping lurid stories about what had supposedly happened. One version doing the rounds was that I had stripped off in a lift and made a lunge at Glenys Kinnock. Another that I had been arrested after going up to the top table at the dinner, downing every single glass there and collapsing in a heap. So it was all over. And then it wasn't. Because of that call from 'Stotty'.

In the hospital, picking up the pieces from my breakdown, I had my first experience of psychiatry not for Donald but for myself. Dr Ernest Bennie had a calm, quiet voice, and his being Scottish helped put me at ease. He didn't mind silence. He was happy to wait for answers.

Amid the possessions I had chucked on the floor of the council building in Hamilton, now returned by the police, was my A4 diary.

'I notice you keep a diary,' said Dr Bennie.

'I do.'

'Why do you do that?'

'To record what I do with my life.'

'And why do you do that?'

'I don't know, I always have.'

'When did you start doing that?'

'I have always written a lot. I used to write match reports of football matches I went to. I wrote to relatives in Scotland telling them what was happening in school. And when my Dad was in hospital after his accident, we couldn't visit that often, so I sent him letters with my Mum every day. They were just accounts of my day. I think that is when the habit started.'

'And let me ask you this . . . in your diary, would you ever make a note of how much you drink?'

'No. Why would I do that?'

'I don't know.'

Silence.

More silence.

'Do you think I should?' I ask.

'Should what?'

'Record my drinking.'

'I don't know. I just wondered if you did.'

Silence.

'No. But I could if you wanted me to.'

'I wonder if we might take a few recent days, and try to track back, and establish whether you can recall how much you were drinking? Do you think you could do that?'

'I suppose so.'

'You will have to read to me. I can't read a word of your writing.' My diaries are a mix of longhand and shorthand micro-scribbles and the entries were especially micro in the run-up to my breakdown.

'Try that day,' he said, as I flicked to an especially manic-looking Tuesday.

'Woke up. Waited for F to go swimming. Went to the toilet. Threw up. Fuck! This is happening too often.'

'What is happening too often?'

'Throwing up in the morning. I think that is what I mean.'

Silence.

'Go on.'

'Into work. Meeting with Tony Holden [editor]. Still not hired enough staff but budget smashed. Briefed

Geordie Greig [reporter] on a few ideas. Conference.
To the Lord High Admiral . . .'

'Which is?'

'The office pub.'

'I see. What time might this be?'

'About eleven. Just after maybe.'

Silence.

'Carry on.'

'Back for a meeting, then back to LHA before going
for lunch with David Mellor.'

'The politician?'

'Yes. Then it is just stuff about what we talked about
– football, Thatcher blah, Nigel Lawson blah.'

'And did you drink over lunch?'

'Mmmm.'

'Wine?'

'Yes.'

'Much?'

'Maybe a couple of bottles.'

'Mmmm. Go on.'

'Then back to the office. Then a meeting in
Vagabonds.'

'Vagabonds?'

'A drinking club.'

'I see. What time are we now?'

'Three-ish, maybe half-three.'

'And what would you be drinking there?'

'Usually half pints and Scotch chasers.'

'How many?'

'A few.'

'Go on . . .'

But I didn't need to. I'd got the point. A very large penny was dropping in my head.

He made me go on anyway, to the after work session in the pub, several pints of beer and then onto Scotch again, and home around midnight for another row.

He left me with my thoughts, and when he came back the next day, I said to him I was going to try to stop drinking. And I did.

Later, another great and loyal friend, *Mirror* colleague Syd Young, with whom I stayed in the West Country for a while after leaving hospital because I was too fragile for London, brokered my return to the *Mirror*. He arranged for me to meet Richard Stott in a pub – this was at Richard's insistence, he wanted to see I could survive a couple of hours in a bar without being tempted by booze – and we agreed that I would start at the bottom again, on less money than I was on when I left, certainly much less than I was on at *Today*, and I would do night shifts for the first few weeks back. It might sound harsh. It wasn't. It was the second time in my life – the first when he erroneously offered me the six weeks of shifts – that he had given me a massive break. Even writing this now, I can feel that burden rising from my shoulders once more. I felt valued, and respected for abilities he saw as being undimmed, even by psychosis. Just as Glasgow University would not define Donald by his illness, Richard would not define me by mine. He was willing to take a risk on me. It was a trust I never forgot, and always treasured and honoured.

And my other friends continued to look out for me. As, for instance, my first story on my first day back at the *Mirror* was the breaking news of a terrorism incident at Heathrow airport, the location that had played a big part in my recent meltdown. Even as the tube train sped to the airport, I was starting to panic. By the time I got there, I could barely function. I felt sick, anxious, scared. I called Syd from a phone box. He talked me through what I needed to do but then, realising I probably couldn't go through with it, ended up basically doing the story for me, from his house in Somerset, where he was 'our man in Bristol'.

This helped me get my nerve back and it was not long before I was back on the day shift, doing the big stories again, and not long after that I was being promoted, eventually to political editor. Then I followed Richard to a very different, left of centre *Today*, which is where I was when Tony Blair became leader of the Labour Party and asked me to work for him. And this time Richard understood and made no effort to stop me. He was a great man, and that phone call to Ross Hall Hospital one of the greatest acts of kindness – and greatest strokes of luck – I ever experienced. How many other editors might have preferred to bask in the knowledge they had been proved right, and leave me to wallow in my own misery?

7

POLITICS

There had been a lot of politics in my breakdown. Perhaps that is inevitable, in that there has always been a lot of politics in my life, and in my head. At university my views were certainly anti-establishment, and very anti the class-bound nature of British society, but they were ill-formed, and it was only really when I became a journalist that I realised most of the things I believed put me very firmly in the political box marked Labour. I have been there ever since, even after being expelled for voting tactically for the Liberal Democrats in the 2019 European elections in protest at Labour's stance on Brexit.

That sense of Labour being my home was strengthened by living for a while with Fiona's very Labour parents when we first moved to London, and then by the friendship I had forged with Neil Kinnock, before I had become a political reporter. Perhaps it was fitting that he was there on the day I cracked.

When my psychosis-induced paranoia was in full flow, I couldn't hear the words 'left' or 'right' without acute anxiety about their political context, real or imagined. Road signs that instructed me to 'keep left' or said 'right turn only' were enough to provoke real panic that both had to be, and yet could not be, obeyed. On the day of my breakdown I drove round a round-about dozens of times, before realising I was in no fit state to drive, dumping my hire car in Rosyth Naval Dockyard. I wonder if I kept going round and round because it meant I didn't have to choose between going left or right.

Post arrest, at Hamilton police station, when a kindly officer asked me if I was 'all right', I imagined he was asking me if I had shifted my politics to the right, as in 'totally right-wing', and I snarled that there was no way he was going to get me to shift towards Margaret Thatcher. Unsurprisingly, he looked rather perturbed at this, and went off to check whether the duty doctor had arrived yet.

He had already clocked that I was not of terribly sound mind, because when he asked on my arrival whether he could get me a drink, I had imagined I was not in a cell but a cocktail bar: 'I would like a bottle of your finest champagne, my man.'

'I think Irn-Bru is about the fizziest we've got,' he replied, good-naturedly.

Once the doctor did arrive, I was taken to a different room for examination, and he asked me to give him my left hand so that he could take my pulse. My mind went into overdrive, suspicious that his request was also part of the ongoing plot to get me to become a Tory.

'Why left?'

'Pardon?'

'Why my left hand?'

'Because it's nearer to me than your right hand.'

'So, left is OK?'

'What do you mean?'

'You know exactly what I mean.'

'OK. Do you mind if I take your blood pressure? Which arm would you prefer to use?'

'Left.' Pause. 'Was that the right answer?'

'Pardon?'

'Right. As in correct. If right is correct, is left wrong?'

Little wonder that after consultation with the police officers, he decided I could leave, on condition I agreed to go to hospital.

The colours red and blue also created zinging pangs inside my head. Perhaps it was the fact I was wearing a red tie – as I often did – that made me start to divest myself of clothes and possessions in the council building where I was cracking up, beginning to worry I was being challenged in a fight for survival.

Once I was in the cells, I began to wonder whether the reason police officers were sometimes called 'the boys in blue' had less to do with the colour of uniforms than a sinister relationship with the Tories. It suddenly crossed my racing mind that I had left the *Mirror*, with its famous red masthead, for *Today*, whose masthead was to be blue. Perhaps I had fallen victim to some elaborate right-wing plot? Operation Masthead – Red to Blue. Was this imprisonment central to it?

This aspect of the madness continued for some time. A few days later, at Ross Hall Hospital, when I had been stabilised through rest and medication, the nurses suggested to Fiona that we go for a walk outside so that I could get some fresh air for the first time since my arrival. It seemed like a good idea at the time. However, shortly after leaving the hospital, we entered a small park, and I noticed that to my left there was a row of blue barriers, and to my right there was a red shed. Panic . . . 'blue to the left, red to the right, what the fuck is going on? . . . the world order is being turned upside down . . .' and I said to Fiona, 'I can't do this, we have to go back.'

'Come on,' she said, 'you'll be all *right*.'

Aaargh . . . she is in on it too!!!

It does leave me wondering: if there was so much politics in my madness, was it partly politics that drove me mad?

Certainly, there had been a political dimension to my leaving the *Daily Mirror*, a Labour paper totally in tune with my views, to join Eddy Shah's *Today*, which had been born in part out of the ongoing attempt by right-wing media owners, notably Rupert Murdoch, to break the hold of the trade unions on the workings of the newspaper industry.

Even though *Today* was not going to join the Murdoch papers in being aggressively pro-Tory, nor was it going to be pro-Labour, and part of the discomfort I felt from day one in my new role as its news editor was the need to engage in a near permanent struggle to make sure the paper did not drift too far to the right.

Indeed, the reason I was on the road with Neil Kinnock on the day of my breakdown, days ahead of the paper's actual launch, when perhaps I should have been in the office, was my determination to ensure a prominent Labour voice in the first edition.

Neil, suspicious of Shah's paper from the off, had insisted that if he was going to do an interview, it would only be with me. Just as he would later warn me against working for Tony Blair, saying it would ruin my life and put our young family under massive strain, so he had warned me against leaving the *Mirror*. On balance, I think I was right to ignore him in working for Tony, but wrong about going to *Today*, even if the breakdown proved helpful in the end in forcing me to sort myself out.

By the time Tony became leader of the Labour Party following John Smith's death in 1994, the crack-up was almost a decade behind me, I had not touched a drop of alcohol in all that time, and although the depressions still came and went, I had kept in pretty good shape. Fiona and I had stayed together despite my provocations, and we had two wonderful sons and a recently arrived, beautiful baby daughter. I had rebuilt my career, first at the *Mirror* under Richard Stott, then at the *Sunday Mirror* as a political reporter and later political editor, then back at the *Mirror* as political editor.

I was also becoming a regular presenter and commentator on TV and radio. By the time I was forced out of the *Mirror* by new management, Richard was editor of a revamped *Today*, which, surprisingly, he was being allowed to make the most pro-Labour paper in Murdoch's stable, where it now resided. So at his invitation I joined as assistant editor in charge of politics.

Yet, when Tony first asked me to work for him, the breakdown returned to the front of my mind. I said 'No' many times before saying 'Yes'. I had cracked up under pressure before, and even though I had made important lifestyle changes, I knew the pressure at the sharp end of politics would be far greater than anything I had ever experienced in newspapers.

Inevitably, a part of me was asking: 'What if I crack up again? And how much damage might I do to the cause I believe in if I do so?' What with the passionate opposition of my family and most of my friends, some of whom likewise worried that the role on offer would play havoc with my obsessive personality and put every-thing I had worked so hard to create – health, welfare, family – at risk, I felt considerable pressure to reject Tony's overtures. Telling him I would 'think about it', I was glad to be able to head to Provence on holiday with my family, and with the Kinnocks.

However, in common with most people who reach the very top, Tony has both the determination to get what he wants, and an instinct about what he needs to do to get it. That instinct told him to change his own holiday plans. He was a few hours to the west of where we were, and a few days later he called to say he would like to join us. So he arrived the next day with his wife Cherie, children Euan, Nicky and Kathryn, and mother-in-law Gale Booth all in tow.

By then, I was already feeling that I might regret passing up this opportunity for the rest of my life and blame myself if Labour ended up losing the next election. Though an atheist, I am still capable of A-grade Catholic guilt.

Two scenarios ran through my head repeatedly during the long sleepless nights as I agonised, knowing that Fiona, peacefully sleeping alongside me, was hoping I would say no.

In one, Tony was standing on the steps of Number 10, waving to the crowds having won a majority, and I was in the press pen opposite, thinking 'I could have been part of that'. In the other, John Major was standing there, re-elected as Prime Minister, waving to very different crowds, and I was in the press pen again, thinking 'I wonder if I could have helped stop that from happening'.

The second image was playing on my mind more strongly. I had written hundreds of thousands of words about why we needed to get rid of the Tories. Now I had the chance to make it happen. By the time Tony and family pitched up, he was pushing at an open door.

It didn't prevent a few 'holiday from hell' days, in which Fiona and Neil tried to talk me out of it in one room, while Tony and Cherie tried to talk me into it in another, with Glenys Kinnock playing a more neutral 'let him make up his own mind and let's support him whatever he decides' role.

In the Fiona/Neil room, the chat would go like this:

NEIL: You will hate dealing with all the wankers you'll have to deal with.

FIONA: Neil knows what he is talking about. He knows you, and he knows more than anyone what the job entails.

ME: But do we want Labour to win or not?

NEIL: Of course.

FIONA: Yes, but why you?

ME: Who else then?

NEIL: There are always people.

ME: But I know I can make a difference.

FIONA: You'll make yourself ill, you know you will.

ME: Why?

FIONA: Because you always do.

ME: No I don't.

NEIL: Listen to her, Ali. They are thinking about themselves. She is thinking about you.

Then, in the Tony/Cherie room:

ME: Fiona is really worried about it.

TONY: Of course she is. It's a big deal. But do you want to change the world or not?

CHERIE: There is only so much you can do as a journalist.

TONY: This is more than press secretary I am
asking you to be here. A lot more. You and I run
the whole strategy, the whole show.

ME: But I've got my life back on track.

TONY: Exactly, and this is made for you. Nobody
else can do this like you can. I know that.

It is not easy to say no to this kind of thing, even if the
reasons for him saying it were so transparent.

When finally I decided I would do it, I also decided
to share the full details of my breakdown with Tony,
along with my concerns it might happen again, given
the pressures I was signing up for. I volunteered to
drive Cherie's mum to Marseille airport for her flight
home, powered partly by my desire to get away from
the two-way lobbying pressures. And Tony immediately said he would come with me.

We had known each other ever since he had become
an MP, so he was aware I had had a breakdown, aware
too that I had had issues with alcohol, and that my
moods could be volatile. But I said he needed to understand just how bad the breakdown had been, and also
understand my concerns at taking the position he was
asking me to, given my continuing occasional struggles
with depression.

Once we had dropped off Cherie's mum and we
were heading back to the house, I tweaked the rear-
view mirror so I could see part of his face as we spoke.
When I got onto the moment of psychotic meltdown,
and the bit where in different parts of my head I could

hear bagpipes, brass bands, football commentaries, Abba, Elvis, a row at work, a row at home, it is fair to say his face took on the wide-eyed contours of what we used to call his 'Bambi look'.

But then he said: 'Well, I'm not bothered if you're not bothered.'

'What if I'm bothered?'

'I'm still not bothered,' he replied.

Just as Richard Stott had refused to define me by my breakdown or broader mental health issues, now Tony Blair, the man likely to become the next Prime Minister, was doing the same. The last hurdle had fallen. The next conversation I had with Fiona was not an easy one, though I think by then she knew which way I was heading.

FIONA: Are you sure?

ME: Yes, I am.

FIONA: And have you thought about us, or just about you, and Tony?

ME: I've thought about Labour, and I've thought about winning, and I know I can help.

FIONA: We have three young children, have you thought about how this changes things for them?

ME: I have, but I think we can manage.

FIONA: Well, I am not sure we can. But on your own head be it.

Many times in the years that followed, through rows, scandals and crises, eighteen-hour days and incessantly interrupted nights, weekends and holidays, I had cause to wonder whether she and Neil Kinnock had been right. I was often unhappy, and almost always stressed, to the point where my own GP once warned me, as I struggled with chest and stomach ailments that he believed were as much caused by mental as physical factors, that I might be underestimating the long-term damage I was doing to myself.

Yet for all the moments of stress, unhappiness, pressure and depression, if I had my time all over again, even knowing what I now know, I think I would do it again. I am happy that I did it, and happy that I made a difference. The whole experience has strengthened my belief that happiness is less about what we feel in the moment, but how we feel about what we do over time, and that we do not know if we have lived a happy life until we near its end. This may be my atheist's way of staying broadly on the straight and narrow without the belief in or moral guidance of the Man Upstairs so loved by my sister, but I believe it to be true.

It would have been hard to maintain the commitment to the work I did had I not believed in what Tony was trying to do, in the main enjoyed his company and the challenges we worked on, enjoyed working with the team we built and, crucially, felt that I was making a difference. But though Tony started off with that empathetic understanding of my mental state, and often showed it subsequently, he could be a hard taskmaster.

Weekends were particularly difficult. He would phone, and say he was worried about me, that I had seemed stressed and ratty, and he felt I needed to take it easy for the weekend, rest, sleep. Fine, I would say. But then he would run through half a dozen issues on his mind, most of which carried the instruction, sometimes spoken, sometimes understood by me without it being spoken, that I should do something, call this minister or that, square this MP or that, brief this journalist or that, write this speech or that. No rest.

I often saw Tony anxious and worried, sometimes dejected, but never depressed. He generally has a very sunny disposition towards the world, even when it seems not to be turning in his favour. That lack of personal experience of depression might explain the somewhat cavalier attitude he displayed to mental illness in his autobiography, *The Journey*, which led to one of my very rare public criticisms of him.

I did not object to his reference to me as a 'rock', and even less did I complain at his over the top description of me as a 'genius'. Where I took umbrage was when he referred to my mental health issues, and wrote: 'In my experience there are two types of crazy people: those who are just crazy, and who are therefore dangerous; and those whose craziness lends them creativity, strength, ingenuity and verve. Alastair was of the latter sort . . .'

So he goes on, culminating a few hundred pages later with his view that if I had still been around in his final days as Prime Minister, when the media had become even more ludicrous, I would have rampaged around like 'a mad axeman'.

Friends and fellow campaigners urged me to say something, so I did, writing a piece, which I sent to him to make sure he saw it, in which I argued that this kind of thinking played into, rather than challenged, the stereotypes we have been working hard to break down.

The stereotype runs something like this – 'if you are crazy, you can either be a creative genius, or you're likely to be a menace to society, running around stabbing people to death because Jesus told you to'. But the reality is most people with mental health problems are neither. They are ordinary people leading ordinary lives, capable of making a contribution but not always allowed to, and far more likely to be victims of violence than perpetrators. Rare slap on the wrist for TB, over. He took it well at the time.

When the depressive episodes struck in Number 10, mostly, I just got on with it. I have always had a strong work ethic and a low boredom threshold. I have for the most part been blessed with high energy levels, and provided I can see the purpose of a course of action, and believe in it, I am motivated to pursue it to the end.

The worst times were when my political and personal lives collided, as when Fiona and I argued over policy, especially Iraq, or when I was forced to work hard and long hours to promote policies which did not excite or inspire me, or defend the personal conduct of others that I didn't support – such as some of the education choices some of our team made for their own children or when ministers did really stupid things, either politically or in their personal lives.

Only once, so far as I can recall, did my mental health lead me not to do something that I normally would have done. A depressive cloud had come in overnight. Six and a half out of ten maybe; the blind on the landing stayed down. I forced myself to run to work, thinking it might help chase the depression away. Instead, all it did was drain me of what little energy I had. By the time I reached the office, showered and dressed, I was exhausted, and felt desperate to get home again. I saw TB as usual, took my morning team meetings as usual, but as I prepared to do the daily eleven o'clock morning briefing in the basement of Number 10, at around ten to eleven, the cloud had become so dark I could not face leaving my office. I called in my deputy, Godric Smith, and said he would have to stand in for me.

GODRIC: Are you OK?
ME: Not really. Feeling really shit.
GODRIC: I'm really sorry.
ME: I'm sorry to land you with this.

Then he told me he had a sister with a serious mental health condition, so he knew all about troubles of the mind. It is remarkable how often, when first being open with someone about mental ill health, you find they have their own story, or that of a family member, to tell.

Mainly, I would tough out the plunges. But I knew intensely when I was not on form, and I knew that others knew it too. Another member of my team, Hilary Coffman, was very good at spotting the signs when my dark mood might take me to excessive irritation with the journalists in briefings, and sometimes anger. Her raised eyebrow and accompanying smile were often enough to deflect me back onto the right path.

My PA, Alison Blackshaw, likewise became very good as a gatekeeper, knowing, and deciding, that most of those who insisted they needed to see or speak to me, actually didn't. On those days I locked myself away, got on with paperwork and avoided the world, and she found little ways of keeping it at bay. 'He's on a call, can't be disturbed . . . he's talking to the PM . . . he's got someone in with him . . .' Fiona, the children and Tony were the only ones she knew she absolutely had to put through if they called.

The key to being able to keep going, though, is resilience. I believe I owe mine in part to my earlier breakdown. A profile writer once said of me that I had had a successful career 'despite a history of mental ill health'. When next I saw him, I thanked him but pointed out that he could, should even, have perhaps changed 'despite' to 'in part because of'.

Resilience is helped by my having a thick skin, something definitely required in politics, all the more so since the advent of social media. It is important to decide whose opinion matters to you, and not be ashamed to hold that your own opinion of yourself matters a great deal.

I consider myself to be a reasonable judge of myself, provided I have others I trust to test my judgement against. At work, Tony's opinion mattered the most. As did that of other ministers and MPs, some more than others. As did that of my team, at all levels. Provided Tony, most of the Cabinet and the Parliamentary Labour Party, most of my team and senior colleagues felt I was doing the job well, that was enough. What the press or the Tories said didn't trouble me, unless it troubled any or all of the above, or when it got to my family, especially my Mum.

Outside work, the only views that mattered to me were those of Fiona and the children, our broader family, and a small number of friends. My trips to Burnley games were also a useful barometer to check out mood and opinion among a variety of people. But had I worried too much about what journalists thought, wrote and said, or the opinions of random members of the public they influenced, most days I wouldn't have bothered to open the bedroom curtains, let alone raise the blind on the landing.

The fact that shortly after leaving my job in Number 10, I had one of the worst and longest depressive episodes of my life, suggests that perhaps I had been keeping depression at bay through a mix of willpower and just being so busy. But politics is in many ways something of a laboratory for mental ill health. It is compelling evidence of the continuing stigma attached to mental illness that just a handful of MPs will admit to having struggled themselves.

Take the life of the average hard-working MP, and you quickly get a sense of why many might struggle: often living apart from family; long hours; most weekends not your own; it's no guaranteed route to wealth; huge demands from large numbers of people who all expect you to be able to resolve their problems immediately; general opprobrium – 'all politicians are useless/in it for themselves/all the same' (all three largely untrue) – and a lot of specific opprobrium too; scrutiny not just of political life but personal life too, past and present; job insecurity. Most MPs do not have as much power as they think they should, or their voters think they do; and those who do have real power find their actions, words, motivations, friendships, holidays, all aspects of their lives subject to scrutiny most would not be able to endure let alone enjoy. It might explain why so few good people now think of going into politics, which in turn might explain why it is currently such a mess.

Politics is really no different to any other walk of life in which people are doing their best to do a job. The big differences are the levels of scrutiny, the significance of the issues under debate and the decisions being made. At heart, like other walks of life, it is about people and their relationships.

There were many strands to my job working for Tony Blair, from the briefings of the Westminster-based journalists twice a day, to broader media management, political management, event management and coordination across government, crisis management, diplomacy, speech-writing, diary planning, lightning conducting, personal and political advice to him and his colleagues 24/7, strategy development and execution. The last of these was the most important, but the hardest, in terms of impact on my mental health, was none of the above.

It was dealing with the fall-outs, the spats, the personalities. There are few things more frustrating than knowing that people can work together – because you have seen them do so, to great effect – and then see them failing to do so properly.

When Tony and Gordon Brown were on song together, and Peter Mandelson and I were working together well, the whole operation was so much stronger. When we weren't, it could be a nightmare. When we were in Opposition, prior to shadow cabinet meetings, we had a meeting that was listed in Tony's schedule as 'Big Guns' – the quartet of Tony, Gordon, John Prescott and Robin Cook. I, always, and Jonathan Powell, often, also attended. Sometimes, these were fine – productive, reasonable meetings, with four very different but very smart and committed politicians thrashing out issues and ironing out problems before taking them to the broader shadow ministerial team. Other times, they could be truly awful.

On a good day, one of the four would not be speaking to another of the four. On a bad day, there would be a sense of animosity, or political divergence, between at least three, occasionally all four, though Tony usually managed to be the most even-tempered, but even he too could lose it at times.

It was not always like this, but when it was, it often fell to me to try to pick up the pieces. I sometimes felt 'Ambassador to JP, Ambassador to GB, Ambassador to

RC' should have been added to the list of my duties above. Internally, and latterly externally in parts of the media too, the difficulties between Tony and Gordon became known as TBGBs (said with the same tone as 'heebie-jeebies', which is what from time to time they gave us). Yet even when the TBGBs were dire, I tried and usually succeeded in having some kind of contact with Gordon. When John Prescott was offside with Tony, it often fell to me to try to get him back onside, and the same, though less frequently, also went for Robin Cook.

Once we were in government, the TBGBs got more extreme: better at times, much worse at others, sometimes unspeakably so – literally, when they were not speaking in a manner most would understand as speaking – and again I was often the emissary between them. This was a role I had shared variously with the Chief Whip Donald Dewar when we were in Opposition, with senior civil servant Jeremy Heywood in government and on the GB side with Ed Balls and latterly Ed Miliband, who was known as 'the Emissary from Planet Fuck', on account of the fact, as TB said, 'he is the only one who doesn't swear at me'. Once we set up broader planning meetings to try to improve things, involving Philip Gould and Douglas Alexander, Douglas and I, both football fans, started calling it 'the Group of Death'.

It says something for our sense of commitment to each other, and to Labour, that despite it all, when Tony finally left, in part pushed out by Gordon, we nonetheless helped Gordon (who could be a nightmare, but was also brilliant) both to take over as Labour leader and Prime Minister, and to fight the election in 2010.

Many friends and colleagues, who knew the background, found this hard to understand. Gordon and I had had some major differences in our time, and said harsh words too, and once I left in 2003, I was hoping the TBGBs were behind me.

But if anything they became an even bigger part of my life, because now I was no longer doing all the other things, I was constantly being buffeted between the two of them. And, despite the history, when Gordon became Prime Minister, he put me under immense pressure, up to and including the offer of a peerage and a Cabinet post, to work for and with him.

My psychiatrist, to whom I confided the huge conflict I felt within myself – part of me wanted to walk away, part of me felt a real sense of duty to help – could not believe I was allowing myself to be drawn back into the world I had been trying to escape. But then – and I write this having been drawn fully into the ultimately unsucessful People's Vote campaign to get a second referendum on Brexit – maybe I wasn't really trying to escape at all. Perhaps the need to be central and feel relevant is another addiction, and maybe politics feeds that more than anything else. It might explain why, although I can say from experience that politics probably has a higher proportion of mentally unstable and psychologically challenged people than other walks of life, so few are willing to admit to it. I think they, and the country, would be a lot healthier if they did.

8

FIONA

My greatest stroke of luck is Fiona. I am lucky beyond belief that I met her, that we fell in love in days, that we set up home in weeks, that she became pregnant a year after my breakdown and we have three of the best and most interesting – and yes, challenging at times – children any parent could wish for.

When she walked into my hospital room in 1986, with her wonderful father, Bob, a yard or two behind, and she said with a smile 'oh Ali, what have you gone and done now?' I knew she was standing by me, when I had convinced myself she wouldn't. Just as I had thought my career was over, so I thought the key relationship in my life was over. I burst into tears of love and relief.

We have had many ups and downs since that day, especially when, against her wishes, I agreed to work for Tony Blair, which did, as she argued it would, take over our lives, put huge pressure on the family and on my mental health, and hers too. There have been times it has been touch and go, times we have talked about breaking up, one time when I asked our eldest child Rory if he thought he, Calum and Grace would be happier if we split (thankfully, he said 'No, definitely not').

Today, forty years after we first met, I enjoy Fiona's company more than I have ever done; which is a good job because we spend more time together than we have ever done, and more than any other non-retired couple I know.

We both work from home. I like being with her. I like talking to her. There is no professional decision large or small I don't share with her. There is no situation large or small in which I would not need and want her judgement – even if I don't always take it. We get on each other's nerves – as all couples do – and can still have the occasional flare-up and meltdown, but so much less frequently than we did.

And when we celebrated her sixtieth birthday in the Scottish Highlands, and I extravagantly hired Skipinnish to play at the party, I don't think I had ever loved her more. It was a small group of family and our very closest friends: Lindsay Nicholson, Gail Rebuck and Sarah Kennedy, the widows of three much missed close friends – John Merritt, Philip Gould and Charles Kennedy – and David Mills, whose wife Tessa Jowell was confined to bed in a nearby cottage, too ill to attend. Skipinnish's accordion player and composer Angus MacPhail later wrote to me, saying the band had played to crowds in their thousands, but the love in that 'audience of tens' was as powerful as anything he had witnessed at the hundreds of gigs they had done.

I am not the easiest person to live with. My temperament and the logistics of my life make that so. But Fiona is not someone who flakes whenever the going gets tough. And there have been times when it has been really tough, not least in the years after I left Number 10, when she had been sure things would get better as a result of that decision and in many ways they got worse.

We have both said some very harsh things to each other, and sometimes we have meant them. There have definitely been times when I have tested her patience and her endurance to the limit, and times when I have taken her for granted. I think most other women would have reached the 'enough is enough' point a long time ago.

But Fiona is not most people. She is strong, smart, caring, and has got better and better at dealing with my mood swings. She spent years blaming herself for my depressions, and now she knows she shouldn't. It can make her seem hard at times, but she needs to protect herself, and not allow my moods to take her down with me. She calls things as they are. When asked what it was like living with me, she said 'never dull, always challenging, sometimes difficult, but *on balance* I am glad we have stayed together'. On balance, and the rest, so am I.

*

A drab, grey Portakabin is not the most romantic of settings, but that was a venue central to our courtship. It was at the back of the main West of England Newspapers HQ in Plymouth, and the place where most of our formal training took place. The desks were arranged in a U-shape around the Portakabin and as luck would have it, we ended up sitting opposite each other. Fiona was elegant and a bit aloof, not someone likely to run with the crowd.

I also learned on Day One that she had her own car, an added attraction as I didn't drive, and when I learned she had bought the purple Mini with blacked-out windows from comedian Peter Cook, the sense of her London glamour was reinforced. MMU 353 L is the only registration of any car in my life – my current car included – that I can actually remember.

Within days, we were peeling off from the rest of the group and heading off in her car to a beach or out to Dartmoor. Whenever she talks to our children or others about those days, she talks about her impression not just of my heavy drinking and smoking, but my sense of real confidence, a belief that I was definitely going places, that I would command and fill any space that I entered. Fine, but it was not always thus. She and the other trainees had an early experience of my squeamishness when we were given a tour of Devon and Cornwall police forensics department and the sight of a blood-spattered body, a murder victim, had me collapse in front of the woman I was desperate to impress.

When, a few weeks in, we were being sent out to one of several local papers dotted around the West Country, I embarked on a heavy campaign of lobbying the head of the training scheme, Jim Dalrymple, that wherever I was sent, could Fiona please be sent there too? And so, barely a month after meeting, we were flat-hunting together, working together, living together. Nothing could have felt more natural, more right.

Looking back, it is amazing we got together. She has always been a health freak, and has swum at least a mile every day I have known her. She has always taken care over what she eats. I have only once seen her the worse for wear through drink, when as trainee journalists we tried to outdrink the eccentric *Tavistock Times* photographer, Jim Thorington, who had the advantage over us of a lifelong predilection for vast quantities of whisky.

When we met, I was a chain-smoking, hard-drinking, crap-food-eating, exercise-free zone. I smoked in bed, lighting up as soon as I woke up. The very thought now makes me feel ill, yet she put up with it. My drinking was never fully under control, having hit genuinely problematic levels when I was at university. Our children, who have never seen me drunk, look shocked whenever Fiona recalls the times she had to drag me upstairs virtually comatose after another night on the Scotch.

But did I drink because I liked it? – yes – or because I was self-medicating an as yet undiagnosed depression? – probably. And that was the other reason I was surprised Fiona fell for me – I could get very emotional

in drink, very teary, very anxious, paranoid at times.
But I have always turned to her with my worries and my
emotions. Not long before my breakdown, I called her
from a drinking club near the *Mirror*, Vagabonds, and
said there were two men there who were measuring me
up for a coffin. I don't know to this day if they were or
they weren't, but I strongly believed they were, and she
listened to me patiently. She then called my editor, Tony
Holden, told him she was really worried about me, and
could he please send someone to get me out of there,
and get me home.

A few weeks after we met, I remember being in a
pub with her in Plymouth, and starting to cry because
my Mum had told me a relative I rarely saw had cancer.
That cannot be the reason I was crying. There was
something else going on here as the distant relative and
I were just not close enough, but whatever it was I was
drowning it in drink and distraction. But because I had
a huge capacity for alcohol, and amazing powers of
recovery, usually fuelled by hair of the dog, I was functioning perfectly well on the professional level, and this
in a profession – journalism in the 1980s – where you
were considered weird if you didn't drink and smoke
heavily, rather than the other way round.

So for years my depressions came and went unac-
knowledged, by me or anyone else. I would no more
have thought of going to see a doctor than I would have
thought of going to a church to confess my sins. So if I
seemed grumpy at times, that was all it was. 'What do
you mean, am I OK? Of course I am. What are you

talking about, do I think I drink too much? I drink way less than (name the last person we saw drunk and incapable). Stop nagging me. Leave me alone.'

'You always hurt the one you love . . .' Fiona took the brunt of my plunges in those times, especially in the days when I refused to accept that anything was wrong, when I felt dead and alive at the same time. Dead in that I could feel the numbness inside, and had lost the desire to live; alive in that I was still breathing, hearing, seeing, knowing there were things I was supposed to be doing that day.

So if the phone rang I might answer, and struggle my way through the call, then collapse again. I might even have a civilised conversation with someone, who would have no idea anything was wrong, but the effort meant the collapse was even faster once the chat was over.

There are so few people we can actually be ourselves with, totally uninhibited, but with Fiona I would just let the depression rule. If she spoke, I felt no need to reply. A tiny headshake would be as communicative as it got. Looking back, I can see how cruel it must have seemed, and why she was driven to feel it must be something that she was doing wrong, something about her, as the key person in my life yet unable to help me.

One time, I did a live TV interview in the street outside our house, Sky News having sent a camera and a satellite van. The interview went fine, then I came back inside and collapsed onto the sofa.

'How can you be like that one minute, and this the next?'

I didn't answer. I can see now why she would think 'it must be something about me'. My only excuse is that yes, it is in part about Fiona, but in a better way than it might seem, because she is the one person I will allow to see me emotionally naked, stripped down to the core.

Holidays have always been danger zones for me. I try to slow down but initially, at least, I just can't. When I do, something work-related inevitably happens that requires – or I think it does – my undivided attention. Then the family pressures rise with every new phone call or hour spent writing, the rows kick off, the spiral kicks in, the depression deepens, five to six, to seven, to eight to nine.

Holidays are supposed to be such fantastic times for families, and often they have been. But they have also provided some of the most painful memories of my life. I remember sitting on the edge of the bath at the house we used to rent in Puyméras, crying uncontrollably, when Calum walked in on me.

'What's wrong, dad?'

'I don't know. I just don't know.'

Or the time I was lying on the bed, weeping, unable to stop. Fiona had been trying to find out what was wrong, then she went out to the garden where Rory was.

'What's wrong with dad?'

'He wants to kill himself.'

That is hard for anyone to hear. One of the best things I did, when finally I got proper help, was to sit the kids down one by one and explain that far from contributing to my depressions they were three of the few people in my life who somehow always helped.

I sometimes worry I have placed too much of a burden on them, because when I feel myself going into a dive, I seek them out. It doesn't always work. If we end up having a row for whatever reason, the plunge can accelerate. Grace and I, in particular, both have the capacity for switching very speedily from calm and reasonable to ferocious loss of temper. But by and large, most of the time, the kids have been good for me, and I hope I have been – on balance, in the main, as Fiona might put it – good for them!

At least Grace, with her 'why I will never go into politics' show, is getting to make a living out of comedy in part at my expense, and I am very proud of her, especially given the anxiety she has had and still gets. I am likewise very proud of Calum for his six years of sobriety and his stunning professional achievements in major sporting events, and now an important film about disability. And of Rory for turning his love of football, maths, poker and gambling into a successful business enterprise. I hope that they believe we have both been and continue to be good parents. But it has been Fiona who has held it (and us) all together.

Back in the days leading to my breakdown, I took what I now see as her concern as nagging, and as trying to stop me doing the things I felt I needed to do for the job I had taken on.

'I'm worried about you.'

'There is nothing to worry about. I'm fine.'

'Everyone is worried about you.'

'Who?'

'Your friends.'

'Who?'

'All of them.'

'Name names.'

'Neil and Glenys . . . Syd . . . Bob and Audrey . . .'

'They're all mad. It's them you should worry about, not me.'

Until my breakdown, I did not even know who my GP was, and only got to know him because a few weeks after I was let out of hospital, Fiona's jaw locked. When she went to see him, he asked if there had been anything stressful happening in her life, and she broke down and told him about what had happened to me.

Tom Bostock became a friend and confidant – and fierce critic of government policy on Iraq, health reforms and much else besides – as well as a caring and considerate GP. By the time I was working for the government, he was convinced – and given what subsequently emerged regarding blagging and phone-hacking, not unreasonably perhaps – that the press were trying to get hold of my medical records. He kept them in a safe at his house off Finchley Road, which is where I often saw him.

But I was still reluctant to admit I had depression, let alone take medication for it. I had defeated drink on my own. I had got over my breakdown on my own. Or so I told myself. In truth I had benefited from the help and support of a small army of people, and this book can mention only a tiny fraction of a very long list of relatives, friends, colleagues, medical experts and accidental strangers, like the two policemen from Fife, who made recovery possible.

For the time being, however, I was part Superman, capable of doing anything I set my mind to, and part still that young boy on the grassy rock in Tiree. 'This is my problem. I will deal with it. Leave me alone. I'm not depressed, I'm just working too hard. Are you saying I'm crazy? You're the one who's fucking crazy, saying I'm crazy!'

And so the cycles went on, and off, and on, and off, and on. By the time I was in Downing Street, I reasoned that if Tom Bostock was paranoid about the press getting hold of my medical records, surely I was right to avoid admitting to mental illness, let alone taking medication for it, because if it was there in black and white, the press would have a field day.

So the denial went on, and on, and on, until it couldn't go on any more. I needed help, but it took my closest friend, not me, to see it first and push me to get that help.

9

FRIENDSHIP

I know a lot of people. I get on with a lot of people. But I don't have that many close friends. Not friends that I know I can count on one hundred per cent. So my closest friends have always been very important to me. Far more important than the various schools, university or workplaces I met them at. And by and large I have been very lucky in my friendships.

John Bailey was my best friend at Utley Primary School. We came from different backgrounds – me the Scottish vet's son growing up in a nice big house at the top end of town, John the son of a local farmhand. Mum could do a decent impersonation of him, and for the rest of her life, whenever John's name came up, she would mimic his thick West Yorkshire accent – 'eh up, Misses Campb-bell, awreet if 'ah use t'toilet?'

We were definitely seen as a bit of an odd couple. But we could walk and talk for hours, about cabbages and kings, everything and nothing. Our lives have gone in very different directions but we have always stayed in touch. John is still in Keighley, still follows the Cougars rugby league team, has recently retired from his job as a machine tool fitter and has also, incidentally, had his fair share of struggles with depression. So maybe depressives have an instinct for each other, even aged five! He said recently he had no recollection of us ever having had a squabble, let alone a fight, through those primary school years.

I am hopeless at dates but I remember 10 December 1968. I remember having to say goodbye to my friends at Bradford Grammar School mid-term, and walk to the house of friends of my parents, the Davidsons, who were driving us down to Leicester (Mum and Dad having gone ahead to our new, smaller house). Dad had had to sell up his private practice after a horrific accident involving a sow, which attacked him while he was treating its piglets, and get a nine-to-five and much lower-paid job with the Ministry of Agriculture. We knew it was a big deal, for them as well as for me, Donald, Graeme and Liz. And they were probably just as sad about it as we were. But the feeling was we just had to get on with it, make the best of it. The fact I can remember it so vividly suggests I wasn't happy about it, nor confident about making the best of it at all.

I remember the Oxford versus Cambridge rugby match being on the TV when I got to the Davidsons' house. I have hated anything to do with that whole 'varsity match' thing ever since. Why is it even on TV? 'Who cares about the bloody Boat Race?' is an annual shout at the telly. It probably helps explain why I became so chippy, so difficult, frankly so lucky on several occasions not to be kicked out, when I later studied at Cambridge. All I know is I have never watched a rugby varsity match since, and that I can remember the score of that one, Cambridge 9, Oxford 6, like a scar.

My brothers and I started at our new school, City of Leicester Boys, also alma mater to footballers Gary Lineker and Emile Heskey, the very next day. It wasn't easy arriving just before the school broke up for Christmas, walking there together and then being split up and taken to our separate classrooms by the head. Once the other kids heard two of us played the bagpipes, we were all immediately saddled with the same imaginative nickname – Jock! I'm not sure this helped with Graeme's feelings about our Scottishness. As for me, not for the first time, I had the feeling that I was seen as Scottish in England, and English in Scotland, which all added to a sense of not really belonging.

It was a good enough school, with some terrific teachers, good sports facilities, and it gave me the education needed to get to Cambridge, a rare event for them. But I never felt fully connected or accepted in Leicester, a feeling I rather ostentatiously expressed in wearing a blue anorak over my black school uniform in class, keeping it on whatever the temperature, and never, ever, taking off my Burnley scarf, despite the constant entreaties of various teachers and, on one occasion, the head, to do so.

Perhaps because I never really took to Leicester, where I lived from eleven to eighteen, I have kept few friends from that period of my life. It was then that my fondness for my football team became something closer to an obsession, which has remained with me ever since. Similarly, the passion for bagpipes and all things Scottish grew along with the greater distance from the place I always felt was my spiritual homeland. Dad, Donald and I played in the local pipe band in Leicester. Once we improved as players, Dad drove us to Peterborough every Sunday to be taught by Tony Wilson, one of the best players alive, certainly one of the best outside Scotland.

I couldn't wait for the holidays to come, when off I would go to work on my uncle Jim's farm in Moscow, near Kilmarnock, the place where my mother had grown up. Uncle Jim (Caldwell), though a lifelong teetotaller – my Mum's family was by and large abstinent, my Dad's side much less so – taught me to smoke (eventually his own smoking killed him, as Fiona's dad's smoking killed him, and Graeme's killed him), and his farmhands taught me to drink. I loved those summers, and a major part of the reason was not being in Leicester. Sorry, Leicester, it was just about my life then, I am sure it is a great place for most of you, Gary Lineker is a top bloke, hates Brexit and loves football as much as I do, and at least you have won a Premier League title and got Richard III's bones!

My antipathy towards Oxbridge had started at the age of eleven and consequently I did not make the most of Cambridge. My Dad drove me from Leicester, and dropped me at the gates of Gonville & Caius College with a single brown leather suitcase (as I kept telling my children when we drove their tons of belongings to their various places of higher education). Saying goodbye, he thrust into my hand an envelope, which I opened later to discover, wrapped inside a ten-pound note which he recommended I spend on some decent food, the quote from *Hamlet*: 'This above all: to thine own self be true, And it must follow, as the night the day, Thou canst not then be false to any man.' It is a quote I have passed on to my own children when they have left home for college, just as his father had passed it to him when he left Tiree for the mainland to study.

But I didn't take to Cambridge. I was probably too young, certainly too chippy, and though I had worked hard at City Boys to get the three 'A's I needed, I had been drinking too much between school and college, and that drinking trend accelerated.

And, of course, there had been Netley. Donald's illness had changed the way I looked at the world. I was developing a much deeper sense of what was fair and what was unfair, and I took a large dislike to a lot of the people I was now alongside. Though some public schoolboys became friends, far more became enemies. The braying, the toff accents, the dressing up in old school or rowing club blazers, above all the sense of entitlement – I took against it all in a big way. I had never really thought much about the impact of private education on broader society, but now I developed a profound belief that it was one of the greatest drivers of inequality and of the class system, which has held

Britain back. I only wish we had done more to tackle the basic injustice at its heart when Labour was in power. The Etonians are back in charge, for sure.

Back then, however, I was less likely to express my views through political action than by getting drunk in one of the city-centre pubs used by locals rather than students, then going to the College LNB (Late Night Bar) to cause a bit of mayhem. I am not remotely proud of the way I sometimes behaved. It was the kind of behaviour that I would not tolerate from my own children, and would likely challenge today if I saw it in others.

I had a party piece, which was to head-butt juke-boxes, cigarette machines and doors; an encounter with one of the latter required a large number of stitches across both eyebrows, and a round-the-head bandage that I had to wear to a May Ball where I was supposed to be playing the bagpipes (and indeed did, including an after-party duo with jazzman Acker Bilk).

There were good people there, teachers and students, but I was glad when I was able to leave for France for my year off, and even gladder when I graduated and left the place a year later, with a decent degree but no clue what I was going to do with my life. That year abroad, and my slightly more mature attitude to my final year, confirmed my view I had gone to Cambridge too young. I wish I had taken better advantage of the access to intellectual development that was open to me. I remember towards the end of my time there wandering in to a lecture by George Steiner, the American philosopher, and being blown away by how clever he was, how well he explained really complicated issues, and wondering why it had taken me four years to realise there had been chances like this available to me every day I had been there.

I did nonetheless make a small number of close friends, most of whom have remained friends to this day. None of them are in media or politics. Mike Stephens, a fellow linguist, became a singer. Robin Coupland became a doctor who specialised in working in war zones, then gave it all up and became an artist. Another medic, Geoff Hamilton, became a GP in Jersey, and given how he behaved as a student, I hope for the sake of the people of the Channel Islands that he has changed as much as I have. Kevin Jones became a head teacher, Mark Neale a film-maker, Richard Harffey worked in reinsurance before starting his own delicatessen. The one I see the most, Tim who I mentioned earlier, is bipolar and has had serious mental health challenges all his life, and got himself into all manner of scrapes in different parts of the world, some of which I have had to help him out of, including once, to his eternal delight, by involving the secret services.

One of my closest friends at Cambridge, Mark Gault, dropped dead of a heart attack in New York on the day in 2003 that the BBC broadcast the (false) report which led to the suicide of weapons inspector David Kelly, the Hutton Inquiry, and in some ways the chain of events which finally persuaded me it was time to get off the political front line. It was quite a feat to get to, and speak at, Mark's funeral in the States, while all the time trying to handle the fallout from the political storm which had erupted, and prevent the media from finding out where I was. I am rather proud of the fact that one of the best notes I ever sent to TB, which was made public at the Inquiry, was written on the plane to New York after I had penned the eulogy to Mark, full of drinking stories which shocked Mark's sons, Jack and Harry, as much as Fiona's tales of my drinking days had shocked Rory, Calum and Grace.

I can go years without seeing some of the above friends, but when I do, we can pick up where we left off, and stories we have relived so many times before can be happily retold. I also have friends from my days in journalism, friends from my time in politics and many made through my love of sport. But the real significance of friendship is to have a pool of people, in different places, from different walks of life and different stages of your life, with whom you can feel relaxed and have a good time but, more importantly, on whom you can depend. To be a good friend this has to be a two-way thing. I don't mind being leaned on. I can be good in a crisis. I can give clear and honest advice. Maybe it is the depressive coming out in me again, but the real friends are the ones there not just when things are good, but in the bad times too.

10

GRIEF

My father died after a long illness some years ago. The length of the illness did not prepare me for the shock or how it would feel when he died. I felt like I was living in a perpetual fog. In my dreams I kept looking for him and sometimes thought I could see him. Gordon Brown sent me a lovely letter, saying that every day he saw his own father standing in front of him, trying to give him guidance and strength. I still try, and often succeed, to get similar strength and guidance from my own father, his ashes now scattered over the land where he worked as a vet.

Grief has played a major part in my life. I have lost too many friends, not just brothers and cousins, far too soon. I've been to far too many funerals. I reckon I have delivered more eulogies than some vicars – both my parents, both my brothers, Fiona's dad, loads more – carried more coffins than some undertakers and piped at more funerals than I can even recall. These are situations that need such rigid control that I always take diazepam or temazepam beforehand, so my memories can be pretty hazy.

I do remember as we filed out of the church after yet another funeral, that of Phil Bassett, a fellow *Mirror* trainee who had gone on to work for me in Number 10, my Downing Street colleague Anji Hunter saying, 'remind me never to become one of your best friends, Ali – they all seem to die!'

Mark Gault was just 45. John Merritt, my closest friend in journalism, was 35 when leukaemia killed him, and a few years later it killed his daughter Ellie. Despite the drugs, I couldn't even get to the end of the eulogy when I spoke at John's funeral. Alisdair Macdonald, so often 'my' photographer on the *Mirror*, was 67 when he died, an event that led to one of the best books ever written about grief, his daughter's *H is for Hawk*, in which I briefly appear, speaking at his memorial. Charles Kennedy was just 56 when drink finally got the better of him, and I often castigate myself for persuading him to go to the same rehab place that had helped Calum but failing to get him to turn up. Charles agreed, in theory, but didn't see it through in practice. Richard Stott was 64 when he died. Mark Bennett, my assistant in Number 10 who quit the civil service to work for Labour in the 2001 election, and when I left Number 10 came with me to be a researcher and adviser on my diaries and much else, dropped dead at just 44. Cabinet Secretary Jeremy Heywood died aged 56. Henry Hodge, husband of Labour MP Margaret, was 65. Tony Bevins, a journalist hero as well as a friend, was 58 when pneumonia killed him. From the *Mirror*: Phil Mellor, 69; Ted Oliver, 60; Simon Ferrari, 51; Tom Merrin, 62; Frank Palmer, 66;

Barry Wigmore, 65; Bill Kennedy, 71; Peter Stone, 61; James Whitaker, 72; Harry Arnold, 73; Murray Davies, 67; Chris Buckland, 73; Joe Gorrod, 74; and so many more in their sixties and early seventies. Another *Mirror* colleague, and another eulogy: Christine Garbutt, who never recovered psychologically from a horrific rape at her home and died aged 69. Her partner Chris Lander, the *Mirror*'s cricket correspondent and great pal of Ian Botham, went from cancer aged 59. Don Mackay, also of the *Mirror*, died at 63, and my pipes were singing on the day of his funeral, and people danced on tables at the wake, which he would have loved. Labour MP Sean Hughes, great contact and friend when I was on the *Mirror*, died aged 54.

When I jumped careers to politics, Donald Dewar, 63 – now, that was a funeral and a half – Robin Cook, 59; Mo Mowlam, 55. John Smith of course, whose death at 55 led to the biggest change in my professional life when Tony succeeded him. Burnley chairman Frank Teasdale, bachelor, no kids, at least reached his eighties, and I was stunned to be left a generous legacy in his will. The wife, Kath, and then the son, Chris, of ex-manager Stan Ternent died within nine months of each other, aged 70 and just 49. Players who had been heroes when I was growing up, that I got to know: Ralph Coates, 64; Peter Noble, 73.

And Tessa Jowell, one of the nicest politicians ever made, was 71 when a brain tumour took her. She asked me to pipe the Skye Boat Song at her funeral, and I am pleased to say I played that and the laments to lead her coffin from the church to the hearse better than ever before. Even Donald would have had to recognise that, and he was my biggest critic when it came to the pipes, feeling I did not practise enough (as though I had nothing else to do!).

But the friend who has had the greatest impact on my life and who I miss every day is Philip Gould. When he died, I felt I had lost a limb. Years after his death, I would find myself texting him for his thoughts on a problem, or simply to tell him something funny I had heard or observed, and be halfway through tapping out a message before remembering: he's not there.

Philip was far and away my closest friend in politics. From the day we met, we spoke every day, often dozens of times. We went on holiday together with our families, socialised together and went to sporting events together. We had the time of our lives at the Athens Olympics, held the same opinions on most things, but challenged each other all the time. Philip was a very special human being.

Even when he entered what he called 'the death zone', he was constantly asking himself not just how to make things easier for his wife Gail, and their daughters Georgia and Grace, but how in talking about his death he might help others, and what he might write and say that could help the Labour Party in the future. He would be fascinated, astonished, devastated perhaps, to see the state of the Labour Party, and of politics more generally here and in the US, today.

He was a team player, and his team was Labour, as it was mine. He was also great in a crisis, and always able to lift people and campaigns when they were low. He was that rare thing in politics – someone who was strategic, tactical and empathetic all in one. He was a rock.

TB could never understand how Philip and I could spend so much time working together, and go on holiday together as well. The only 'holiday' Tony and I ever had together was the one he gatecrashed to talk me into working for him. For Philip and me, of course, it was partly a way of carrying on working. We shared workaholic tendencies and an obsession with doing all we could to help Labour win and, once we had won the first time, win again. Some of our best strategies, ideas, lines and slogans came from long holiday chats occasionally interrupted by Gail and Fiona asking if 'you two' ever had a conversation that didn't mention TBGB (answer: not many, right to the very end).

Though all too often, for all his capacity for political organisation, he created mayhem by losing passports or wallets or jackets (just as once he lost our entire election plans on a train coming back from one of his focus groups), he was the organiser, the originator of trips and tournaments, madcap events that turned inevitably into holiday highlights.

And when times were tough, there was no better friend – always loyal, but understanding that loyalty required honesty and frankness, and ideas about how to make things better.

When Fiona and I saw him for the last time, we knew we were saying goodbye. It was painful of course, but there was magnificence to it all too. Philip's death was different. He always needed a campaign, and the illness became the campaign. Every campaign needs a simple goal, and he had one – survival. He called the cancer Adolf, perhaps the ultimate enemy. Yes, I said, and this means you are Churchill. He liked that. We had slogans for the fight. He had a grid of his chemo visits, when to take his pills.

Early on in the illness, he told me he had had a PET scan.

'What is a PET scan?' I asked.

'It's like the exit poll,' he said.

'And how is it looking?'

'OK, but all within the margin of error.'

For once, he lost a campaign. He had fought the cancer harder than anyone. But he was reconciled, and he had helped Gail and the girls, and all his friends, to this point too. And he had had a lot of wins along the way. He wrote two books while ill, one on his cancer, which he was working on to the last hours of consciousness, and the other a wonderfully defiant update of his political book, *Unfinished Revolution*, with the basic message that New Labour changed Britain and British politics for the better. We did this in no small measure thanks to Philip.

Philip's politics flowed from deep values and beliefs, which became more spiritual with time. He believed the political elite, including Labour in the wilderness years, had forgotten about lower middle-class families like the one he had come from. He ensured that the voice of ordinary, decent British families was always heard at the top table of British politics. That was the real purpose of focus groups. He saw them not as consumer-led public relations, but as profoundly democratic. Politicians have to lead, of course. But they also have to listen, and nobody was a better political listener than Philip.

Though best known for his focus groups, he involved himself in all aspects of election planning. He was also a brilliant analyser of speech drafts, always offering the kind of frank advice which forced Tony Blair and the speechwriting team to raise our game, as in this entry in my diary for 27 September 1999: 'Philip captured the lowest point around 2 a.m. Tuesday when he did a note which began "this speech has seriously lost the plot. The main argument is nowhere. What has happened?" '

But it is not Philip Gould the strategist, nor Philip Gould the gutsy fighter against cancer that I miss most, but Philip Gould the friend who made our lives better, Philip Gould the positive life force who brought hope and energy to all he did, and Philip Gould the persuader, the man who broke down my resistance to admitting I needed help in defeating my depressions.

There are many ways to judge the people you know. Two important ones for me are how they relate to my children, and what their own children are like. Georgia and Grace are wonderful young women, a tribute to a mother and father who always led busy lives, but who were utterly devoted to their daughters. As for my own children, they loved Philip for the fun, the joy, the support and the friendship he brought into our lives.

Whereas most people who knew and worked with me might easily be aware of my mood swings – I am not the best at hiding them – most who worked with Philip would be unaware that he had very dark moments too. He was much better at putting on a happy face. Unlike me, he saw someone to talk to about his mental health. That someone was David Sturgeon, Philip's psychiatrist. It took him several weeks over one of our holidays to persuade me to go and see him on my return. He booked the appointment for me. I went, not just the once, but dozens and dozens of times thereafter. I had found the right guy for me, thanks to Philip knowing me as well as he did, being the friend that he was and patiently persevering until I was ready to say yes. It was a belated but important step on the road to coming to terms with all that went on in my mind.

Funerals can be such wonderful, healing events, and Philip's, at All Saints church, Margaret Street, in central London, was one such. I had visited the church before because Philip did God more and more as his life neared its end.

'Is this an insurance policy against hell?' I asked, as he insisted I accompany him to his late-in-life Confirmation.

'You'll be there one day,' he said. 'With God, I mean, not hell! The drunk who became teetotal. The anti-psychiatry man who now can't get enough of his shrink and his pills. The anti-exercise fanatic who now does marathons. The dog-hater who became obsessed with his dog. God will get you eventually.' Tony always says his only worry if I do get God is that it will be as an Islamic fundamentalist.

Philip would have loved the beauty of the choir's singing at his funeral, the hymns and readings being sung and read so well, the prayers (read by his sister, one of the first women priests), the incense, the long queues waiting to take Communion. He was not without ego, so he would have also loved the packed church, the photographers outside, the big party afterwards, and the sense of drama and history attached to the event. Two Labour Prime Ministers, Tony and Gordon, in the front row, both doing readings chosen by Philip. Two more Labour leaders, Neil Kinnock and Ed Miliband, behind them. Many key figures of the past Labour government, and the then current coalition government, paying their respects. I know he would have hugely enjoyed the sermon, in which Revd Alan Moses made a compelling case against Tory education policy, with then Education Secretary, Michael Gove, a few pews away, blushing.

I had had an agreement with Philip, having spoken at so many funerals and memorials of relatives and friends before, and always finding it hard, that I wouldn't have to speak at his. But finding him asleep when I went to see him on the day before he died, I wrote him a letter that Georgia and Grace read out to him. When they finished, he smiled and said he wanted it read at the funeral. It was a private letter, but as I ended up reading it in public at his and Gail's request, I thought I would put it in here too, as a tribute not just to Philip, but also to friendship.

Dear Philip,

I hope, as do so many others, that somehow you find within you the strength to carry on. The courage you have shown since the day you were told you had cancer has been inspiring. If anyone can keep on defying the medical odds, you can.

But if this does defeat you this time, I don't want you to go without me saying what a wonderful person you are, and what an extraordinary friend you have been. Of all my friends, you are the one who touches virtually every point of my life – past, present, politics, work, leisure, sport and holidays, education, books, charity, and, more important than anything, family and friendship. I have been blessed to know you. So has Fiona. So have Rory, Calum and Grace. For so many of the happiest moments of our lives, you have been there, indeed often the cause of the happiness.

You've always been there in tough times too. You remember the Alex Ferguson quote – 'the true friend is the one who walks through the door when others are putting on their coats to leave'. You have displayed that brand of friendship so often, so consistently, and with such a force as to keep me going at the lowest of moments.

When I got your moving, lovely message on Tuesday, and was convinced you wouldn't see out the night, I felt like a limb had been wrenched from me. You know my crazy theory that we only know if we have lived a good life as we approach its end – perhaps we only know the real value of a friend when we lose him. The loss for Gail, Georgia and Grace will be enormous. But so many others were touched by you and will share that loss.

My favourite quote of our time in government came not from me or you, or any of the rest of the New Labour team. It came from the Queen in the aftermath of the September 11 attacks ten years ago. 'Grief is the price we pay for love.' You are much loved. There will be much grief. But it is a price worth paying for the joy of having known you, worked with you, laughed with you, cried with you, latterly watched you face death squarely in the eye with the same humility, conviction and concern for others which you have shown in life.

I will always remember you not for the guts in facing cancer, brave though you have been, but for the extraordinary life force you have been in the healthy times. Your enthusiasm, your passion for politics, and belief in its power to do good, your love of Labour, your dedication to the cause and the team – they all have their place in the history that we all wrote together. I loved the defiant tone of your revised *Unfinished Revolution*, your clear message that whatever the critics say, we changed politics and Britain for the better. So often, so many of our people weaken. You never did. You never have. You never would. That is the product of real values, strength of character, and above all integrity of spirit.

In a world divided between givers and takers, you are the ultimate giver. In a world where prima donnas often prosper, you are the ultimate team player. Perhaps alone among the key New Labour people, you have managed to do an amazing job without making enemies. That too is a product of your extraordinary personality, your love of people and your determination always to try to build and heal. It has been humbling to see you, even in these last days and weeks, trying to heal some of the wounds that came with the pressures of power. We can all take lessons from that, and we all should.

Of course I will miss the daily chats, the banter, the unsettled argument about whether QPR are a bigger club than Burnley. More, I'll miss your always being on hand to help me think something through, large or small. But what I will miss more than anything is the life force, the big voice. You have made our lives so much better. You are part of our lives and you will be forever. Because in my life, Philip, you are a bigger force than the death that is about to take you.

Yours ever, AC

In his final months, Philip had talked a lot about the idea of 'a good death'. I felt at the time he was doing little more than keeping up his own spirits, and those of his family and friends. In truth though, it was a good death, or as good as any death might be. Gail spoke later of there being something truly extraordinary about those final minutes they had together, just the four of them. They knew he was going, he had readied himself, and he had readied them.

When she called to tell me he had died, I was at a party to celebrate yet another amazing landmark in the career of Sir Alex Ferguson as Manchester United manager. Alex had hired the modern pipe band, the Red Hot Chilli Pipers, and I had been really looking forward to seeing them perform live. But the moment I saw 'Gail mobile' come up on my phone screen, I knew. She didn't even have to speak, before I started crying.

'Don't cry,' she said. 'I don't know how to describe it, but there was something almost beautiful about it.'

By the time I went back in, the Pipers were in full swing, but the sound of the pipes, at that moment, brought Lachie, and a very different way of dying, vividly to mind.

II

MY SEARCH
FOR A CURE

11

MY PSYCHIATRISTS

'What is the fucking point, David?' I ask my psychiatrist, David Sturgeon, one morning, a couple of hours after waking up with an eight, after three days stuck at seven.

'The point of what?'

'Life.'

'The point of life is to live it.'

He is full of wise words. They do help, sometimes. I certainly feel I have lived a better life since first seeing him, thirteen years ago.

We had been on holiday, in France, and I was having such a bad time that Philip had made me promise to go and see David when we got back. The gaps between my depressions had been getting shorter and shorter, and the intensity of the bouts worse and worse.

So much about psychiatry, as with any relationship, depends on chemistry and trust. I clicked with David on both fronts from the off. After an initial chat, we started with a long written account of my emotional life, which formed the basis for our first sessions.

Those first few months, seeing David weekly, sometimes twice weekly, were often very painful. I felt like my innards were being torn to shreds. I felt like my soul was on an operating table. Fiona came to some of the sessions, and hearing her say some very harsh things about what it was like to live with me was among the greatest of the pains. The children came too, once or twice, so David could involve them and make sure they understood my depressions were not their fault, that indeed they were about the only people who made life worth living when I was rising up my depression scale.

My first experience of psychiatry, with Donald in his military hospital, was OK. Mixed, but OK. My first experience for myself, with Dr Bennie helping me to pick up the pieces from my breakdown, was excellent. When, years later, I tracked him down to the place where he lived in retirement, not least to thank him, he was aware, or at least had suspected, that the person he kept seeing on TV and reading about in the papers was indeed the Alastair Campbell he had been called out to after I arrived from the police station all those years ago.

I told him that his interventions in the ensuing days had been vital, and it was often as much about what he didn't say as what he did.

He smiled. 'Sometimes the successful interventions can be very, very brief, but the patient must make up his own mind, and be ready to do so.'

I have had other experiences, before and since, that simply have not worked. There was a couple at the Maudsley – one male, one female, all very Freudian – who saw me late in 1986 (inspired by my initial success with Dr Bennie) where I didn't even make it to the end of the session. The final straw came when I talked about being arrested, suggesting it might have been because I was seen as a threat to Neil Kinnock – it was the weekend Sweden's left of centre Prime Minister Olof Palme had been assassinated, and security around Neil was tight.

The man and woman team, each sitting in a corner of a large room, clearly saw this as part of the same paranoid nonsense as my being subject to some test for which the price of failure was death.

'What does it say about you that you feel Neil Kinnock and the Special Branch are part of your breakdown?'

'They were.'

'Well, they may have been, we don't know.'

'We do know. I was there. So were they.'

When they started asking if the guy who led me to the phone had made me think bad things about my father, I'd had enough. 'Fuck this for a game of soldiers,' I said, and walked out.

Funnily enough, my GP later told me they had written a 'very insightful analysis of my situation' – though he refused to let me read it. It was also the first time since my breakdown that I felt an inner strength in voicing my own feelings, so perhaps that had been their intention. But somehow I doubted it.

Then there was the man that David sent me to for a new, innovative form of CBT, which involved him endlessly tapping at a laptop as we spoke, and analysing my words in a weird sort of word cloud that I never fully fathomed. He seemed rather excited to meet me, and worried that prying eyes might pick up on our email exchanges, so he gave me a code name – wait for it – Abraham Lincoln.

'I don't think this is going to work,' I texted David the moment I left. I persevered for a few weeks, but it wasn't working for me. But I know it has been a life-saver for others, so I am not knocking it. And I have done a successful form of CBT (Cognitive Behavioural Therapy) since with David, turning negative thought patterns into positive ones, and finding coping strategies to address behaviours that may do me harm and deal with feelings that drag me down. So maybe it was just a personal reaction.

Once you get the chemistry and the trust with a medical practitioner it is quite something. This person, a week earlier, was a total stranger; and now you are answering his questions about love, hate, sex, power, pain, demons and dreams. So you have to find the right one for you and trust them.

You also have to be prepared to work hard. David has definitely worked me hard. I channelled a lot of the agonies and exercises into my first novel, *All in the Mind*, which is about the relationship between a psychiatrist and his patients and the slow uncovering of the fact that the shrink is as sick as his patients. I don't think David is totally like Martin Sturrock but, when I sent him the first draft, he not only didn't object that the first four letters of their surnames were identical but he even suggested Sturrock's rather grisly fate.

David doesn't claim to know everything. He admits that he can only really work on trial and error. I had been on and off all sorts of medication before arriving a few years ago at something that seems to work, a daily 100 milligram dose of sertraline. (Don't look up the side effects online. You'd never take it if you thought half of them were likely to happen.)

But I still get dreadful plunges, and in recent months he has been trying to get me to take a mood stabiliser normally used to treaty epilepsy. I am so far resisting. But I usually give in, in the end. He usually turns out to be right.

At his suggestion, Fiona and I were very deliberately doing something new and different every week, and one particular week, we went for a boat trip down the Thames to the Maritime Museum at Greenwich, to have lunch, then come back. It should have been a straightforward nice day out. But recently he reminded me that the whole experience plunged me into a terrible gloom, so that on the return journey, I had to lie down on the upper deck seats. What was my problem? I asked him. 'You felt you had achieved nothing in your life compared with Nelson. This is the demon . . . if you are not achieving great things, when you are down, you are very down, and quickly feel worthless. It is awful for you, and awful for the family.'

I had had no memory of any issue with Nelson. Though it reduced us both to near hysterics, David was keen I understand the serious point behind this. He believed it fed into the 'Why him, why not you?' factor regarding my brother Donald. 'You became the star of your family, but you still have this deep, deep sense of not being good enough and when you get depressed that's what really features; you're not good enough, nothing is good enough, and that's what you took away from the Maritime Museum – that you're not good enough, you're not as good as Nelson.' This', he added gently, 'is not what most people do when they go to Greenwich!'

Once, I asked him if he ever thought of his patients when he was just at home, pottering about.

'Only you,' he said.

'Really?'

'Well, you're the only one of my patients that they talk about on the radio. I think about you then . . . but only then.'

I have seen him less in the last two years than I have in any of the previous ten or eleven, so between us we have definitely done something right. Good job I see less of him really. His day job is with students at University College London, and there seems to be an epidemic of anxiety and depression.

But how different might history have been if I had been able to pull off one of his more audacious suggestions.

'I wonder if you shouldn't ask Tony and Gordon if they would mind coming to one of our sessions?' he said, as yet again I spelled out the pressures they were putting me under, and the conflicted feelings those pressures created.

'Not sure that will work,' I laughed.

'No, I'm sure it wouldn't. But it does rather feel like a marriage that is disintegrating.'

'Ah, so you're like a political Relate counsellor now, are you?'

'I can be anything you want me to be, Alastair, anything that is good for you.'

12

DEALING WITH MY DEMON

After my first good conversation with a psychiatrist, Dr Bennie, from being a heavy drinker I stopped drinking just like that. And for thirteen years afterwards I didn't touch a drop. God knows why I decided to try it again – on a whim, at the British Embassy in Bonn in 1999 – but I didn't much like it. I had a sip, swallowed. Had another sip. Spat it out. I do drink sometimes now, but never to excess. David Sturgeon doesn't want me to drink at all, and he is, on this as on so much else, probably right.

Not drinking became my new obsession. I was determined to do it on my own. Unlike my son Calum, now in his sixth year of recovery, I didn't go to Alcoholics Anonymous, though I have since occasionally been to Al-Anon, for families of alcoholics.

The cricketer Geoffrey Boycott, a childhood hero when I was growing up in Yorkshire, became a useful, if unaware, ally. I admired Boycott's dogged approach to run gathering, his refusal to be rushed, his selfishness and his cussedness (I was at this stage unaware of his right-wing views, which might have made me think differently!).

I counted every sober day as one more run, and as I climbed into bed, I would imitate the voices of BBC commentators, first Shipley-born Yorkshireman Jim Laker saying 'there we go, another day, another run, Campbell now on one thousand seven hundred and fifty-two not out. What an innings, Richie.'

'Thank you Jim,' Richie Benaud's lovely Aussie voice would pick up. 'It certainly looks like it is going to take something very special to get Campbell out now.' And so to sleep with a smile on my face. I was well past three thousand runs when I stopped counting.

And yet, and yet, the depressions kept coming, less frequently for sure, especially after we had children, but come they did. That really riled me: I had done the hard bit, I was off the booze, but the depressions the booze had partly hidden were still there and I felt powerless to stop them. A series of various other, possibly healthier addictions kicked in. As Tony Blair once said to Vladimir Putin, when the Russian President noticed I was not touching the various vodkas and wines being lined up as toasts, 'he is not allowed – he is a thing-aholic'. I think Tony would admit he got some benefit from my workaholism, something I still have.

And once my sons got into sport – doing it, not just watching – so did I. The day after my first decent run, in 2002, I entered the London Marathon. I have been an exercise-aholic ever since. I'm a Burnley-aholic. I was a Labour-aholic until they kicked me out for becoming a fully-fledged Anti-Brexit-aholic. I am now something of a mental health-aholic too. This obsessiveness is part of what David calls my demon and – like Fiona – he worries when it kicks in too hard.

David's view is that part of the demon inside me is a desperate desire to be wanted and needed and relevant. Maybe he is right. So when a Prime Minister and a future Prime Minister are pleading with you to go back, the demon rises. Other parts of you know there are dangers. But the conflict burns within me all the time. He said – and I think he is right – that I live in permanent conflict between my concepts of self and service. I want freedom and satisfaction for myself. But I do also want to work with others to change the world for the better. And I think I can.

'That is the demon speaking.'

'But I can. I can do things most other people can't do.'

'The demon speaking. We are all replaceable.'

'Some more than others.'

'Demon.'

We never agree on that one. When I wake up with a two, I think I can reverse Brexit, write a new book in a month and raise half a million quid for a charity. If I am past a six or seven, I think Britain is screwed and there is nothing I or anyone else can do about it. I prefer the two mode.

David worries about the two mode. He worries I get manic, and then the addictive personality kicks in. Not drink addiction, but work addiction, or something I suddenly become obsessed with. This conversation was part of a chat we had for a TV documentary I made.

DS: When the addictive personality trait kicks in, it can be harmful, to you and your family. Back in the day, when you were working with Tony Blair, you were there all the time, you hardly saw your family and they felt very disconnected from you. That was your priority, to do that, and you had to do it well, and you had to do more and more and more of it to keep doing it well. And when you decided to stop doing it, there's this terrible conflict – should I not still be doing it? A terrible sense of guilt, and you have a very powerful sense of duty. You kind of see it as your duty to be there, to do the best that you could. I remember Gordon Brown putting a lot of pressure on you to work for him, to go back into politics and you really got very upset about it because part of you felt you should and part of you felt you shouldn't.

AC: We all have that; everyone has those sorts of conflicts and difficulties.

DS: Not to such an extent. You're a bit special in those regards. But I remember one of your dreams early on when you didn't know what to do with your life, you didn't feel that you knew who you were really and what you should be doing. You had a dream, I don't know if you remember this, in which you felt lost, you were physically lost and you asked an old man to give you directions and he gave you a pen. And you started writing, you started writing novels and in a sense that was a very therapeutic thing for you.

AC: So were you the old man?

DS: I don't know.

I argued that my addictions today are better than those of old, but he was not having it.

DS: That little word 'addict' is like a stick of Brighton rock. The word addict goes all the way through, all the way down, everything that you do; people, places and things, potentially, you can have an addictive relationship with all of them and that's something you have to keep an eye on. It's the demon.

AC: I don't get what you mean by the demon. I get demon drink. But this is different.

DS: It means the addictive part of you – it's like a demon on your shoulder encouraging you, telling you to drink. 'Go on, have another, it'll be all right, you'll feel better.' Of course, you'll feel better, alcohol was your medication, you found something that worked for you. It made you feel like you felt other people were feeling. But it just got – more and more and more.

AC: So what about work? What if the demon is saying, do more work, do more work, get another

job, get another challenge. What's wrong with
that?

DS: Are you going to listen to that? Do you obey
your demons?

AC: I don't know. I think I probably do a lot.

DS: You do a lot. But—

AC: But that's because I like a bit of a challenge or
a bit of a fight.

DS: You do, don't you?

AC: But if I didn't, what would I do? I'd lie in bed
all day?

DS: That's the fear isn't it? The fear is of doing
nothing, of almost being dead.

AC: Being unproductive, unmotivated.

DS: Not doing anything worthwhile.

AC: Why is that not a reasonable fear?

DS: Not a fear that's normal. Most people don't
have that.

AC: They want to do interesting things.

DS: They do. But they tend to do them not to
excess. You go to excess.

AC: And what if you don't want to be most people.
Is that not a reasonable thing to want to be?

I tell him my favourite story about another of my sporting heroes, Sebastian Coe, who is now, after we worked
both against and with each other – against in politics,
with on the London Olympics – a good friend (one
who, incidentally, begged me not to return to politics,
saying I would ruin my life all over again). When Seb

lost the Final he had been expected to win at the Moscow Olympics, and was preparing for the Final he was expected to lose, but in the end won, a sports psychologist told him they needed to create a 'normal environment' to get him in the best possible shape for the race. And Seb, normally placid and mild-mannered, exploded. 'Do you think I'm normal? Do you think what I do is normal? Do you think running three times a day, a hundred miles a week, is normal? I don't. Don't tell me I'm normal. I'm not normal. There's not a single person in this team who's normal. We're all fucking mad.'

When Calum was in the throes of his alcoholism, I found it if anything even harder than my own, because I could see him making the same mistakes and ignoring the same warnings that I had. Watching our own son in the awful slow- then fast-motion descent that alcoholism represents was one of the toughest periods of my and Fiona's lives; and if I had to say why, it was that awful old combination, fear and powerlessness. Fear that he was killing himself. Being powerless to stop him. I remember in the middle of one night, both of us unable to sleep, Calum not home again, Fiona saying: 'Maybe we are just going to have to steel ourselves, that one day there will be a policeman at the door telling us he is dead.'

It felt like that at times, and as often happens with parents dealing with family crisis, though Fiona and I shared the overall objective – try to support him, but try above all to get him the help to stop drinking, he and us so clearly failing on that front – we didn't always agree how. There were times when I would want to be tough, and Fiona soft; other times it was the other way round.

I talked to David about it a lot, because, of course, part of me knew that me being Calum's dad was likely to be an issue, not least when he was working with the Labour Party, and being regularly referred to as 'Alastair's son'; but also because I felt, having had my own troubles with drink, I ought to be able to help him more.

It was partly David who hardened me to an approach best described as 'tough love'. He said Calum would have to hit his own rock bottom before he would begin recovery.

'But what if rock bottom is death? What if he falls in the canal drunk, and drowns? Staggers out in front of a bus? Just destroys his liver anyway?'

'He might. And you won't be able to stop him. You can't be with him twenty-four hours a day.'

Fear. Helplessness.

'So what do we do?'

'You make sure he knows you love him, you care for him, you worry about him. But you set rules, and you keep to them.'

'Like?'

'Like you say he can continue to live with you if he chooses to, but if you find he steals, or lies, or he comes home steaming drunk, you don't let him in.'

'I'm not sure I could do that.'

'You have to.'

'What if I turn him away, and it's the last straw, and he ends it all? Or he wanders off, sleeps rough, dies from the cold?'

'He might, and there is nothing you can do to stop him.'

'But there is: I could let him in.'

'And he would learn there are no rules. He does it again, again, again, the cycle goes on.'

A few weeks later, I was tested almost exactly as we had discussed. Three a.m., tossing and turning. No sign of Calum. No reply to calls and messages. The bell goes. Is this the moment we had been dreading, of the knock on the door from the police?

I go down to the front door, and see Calum slumped against it. I open the door. He has lost his keys. He can barely stand.

'Sorry, Calum, you can't come in.'

'Why not?'

'Because you know the rules.'

'So you're sending me out into the cold for the night?'

'I am.'

I closed the door, slumped against the back of it and, sliding down to the floor, put my head in my hands, and rocked backwards and forwards, weeping.

Calum still has the challenges that created the addiction in the first place, but he has not touched drink since the second of two long spells in residential rehab. He and I still have issues that will need time to resolve. But he is alive; he is incredibly bright, and incredibly hard-working and good at his job. Of my three children, he is still the one likeliest to keep me awake at night, yet I am confident he will get to where he wants to in the end.

13

MIND EXERCISES

I don't know which of the many exercises I have done with David Sturgeon have helped me most. I just know that after a year or two of seeing him I started to feel more hopeful, and generally happier, even if there were many tears and low points along the way, as the innards got turned inside out. No detail was too small for him. It was the same when we got onto my dreams. He wanted all the detail.

Dreams

Once I started recording my dreams at David's request, three possibly related things started to happen. First, I seemed to dream more regularly and more vividly. Second, I remembered them in greater detail when I woke up. Third, sometimes, even as I was dreaming, a part of my conscious mind was making a note to itself, telling me 'you must remember this bit for David'. Sometimes, I found myself waking immediately and, with the dream still fresh in my mind, writing it all down there and then.

David introduced me to 'hypnagogia' and 'hypnopompia', explaining that these are 'twilight state' phenomena which occur when you are either waking up or falling asleep, and so not in clear consciousness. 'You might be half asleep and suddenly hear someone call out your name,' he explains, 'but then you're wondering, "was it a cat?" Or you may feel someone sit on your bed, but when you wake up no one is there. They are very common.'

As to what they mean, it depends on the content, but for a while, when I was recording my dreams every day – it went on for several months, and I sent around 40,000 words worth of them to David for his perusal, amusement and analysis – I seemed to be in this hypnagogic 'lucid dreaming' state quite a lot. Since I have stopped writing down my dreams, I seem to dream less, remember less and have fewer experiences of that twilight state he described.

As to why psychiatrists like to know about dreams, David explained that it was mainly down to Freud. He believed that dreams were a message from the unconscious part of our mind to the conscious part. 'Sometimes it is clear what they mean,' says David. 'We may be reliving some traumatic event from our past, or find ourselves in an anxious situation such as having to give a speech but not having thought about it and standing in front of a roomful of people waiting to hear what we have to say.' He said this kind of thing is almost certainly a manifestation of other anxieties that might be going on in our lives. 'And sometimes we can stop the anxiety by doing something else – such as waking up,' he says.

More often than not though, the dream is not direct, but wrapped up in something else, which he refers to as 'the latent content'. He gave me an example from a young patient. 'He told me of a vivid dream where he was pulling squealing piglets out of a river and being worried about whether they would be all right. His wife was pregnant at the time, and wanted him to be present at the birth, but he was very ambivalent about it.'

As to my own dream log, perhaps one day there is another book in it. It is certainly colourful, and some of it X-rated. When I last read through all the entries, not only had I forgotten the dreams, but in the main I had forgotten the discussions we had about them. How to make sense of something like this, for example?

'I was being shown around a hospital – all a bit edgy and scary – and was taken through an ordinary-looking door into an environment that felt even more edgy. My guide said this was the secure unit. Basically criminal psychopaths, he said, all women. A side door opened and a woman came through in a wheelchair, followed by a female warder. The wheelchair woman was wizened and old. She said, "who the fuck are you and what are you looking at?" Then another woman came through, also in a wheelchair, also with a warder. Grey haired, dirty, menacing. She said nothing. I said to my guide, "I want to get out of here." "No," he said, "stay." I said, "I don't like the atmosphere." The women started to pick up on my anxiety. "What are you scared of? There's nowhere to go." Then they're laughing. I walk through another door and I'm now in a very ordinary house but one wall is like a giant dishwasher and on the other side another patient-prisoner is loading the dishwasher. I now have a child with me, possibly Grace. I say, "come on, let's get out of here". A woman comes through the dishwasher and starts to chase us. I pick up a glass and throw it at her. It doesn't break and just bounces down the corridor. She laughs and carries on chasing us.'

At least there were no 'celebs' in that one. I do recall David pointing out that I was the only patient he had ever had who, in one week's dreams, had Nelson Mandela, Margaret Thatcher and Bill Clinton; Clive Woodward and Arsène Wenger; Anne Robinson and Princess Diana. The fact that I had met them all at some point in my life did not overly impress him. I sensed he felt my mind had gone into Nelson mode again! Nor did the name-dropping stop after his rebuke. In the following week before our next session, Ed Miliband told me I was overweight, and Elton John asked me whether he should have his wedding in Kilkenny or Kildare. I said Kilkenny. The same night, 'Tony, Gordon and I were trapped in the middle of a big crowd of people. It's been announced we have lost the election. They are all cheering and pushing us, hitting us. Security guys move in and have to get us out through a side door. Helicopter waiting, but no pilot! Tony says he has called Barbara Castle. I said Jim Callaghan would be better.' A few days' dreams later, I was working in a bike shop, and the night after that I was working for the Scotland football team on plans to merge with Ireland.

Some of the political ones, save for the odd detail, could just as easily have been real events in my diaries. 'In a tiny room with TB and President Chirac. A spiral staircase goes up from it. We go up. They sit on small wooden chairs very close to each other, opposite, knees almost touching. I am in a more comfortable chair just behind Chirac, wondering who on earth set up this grotty meeting room. They start talking and Chirac is going off on one of his anti-American kicks. He says there is more graffiti in New York than any other city. TB disputes it. Chirac asks me what I think. I say he may well be right but I'm sure we could establish factually the most graffitied city in the world. I get a message to the research department to look for the info. Someone brings in coffee and cakes.'

Here is one you don't need a psychiatry certificate to work out. 'Donald has called me from Aberdeen and says he is in trouble. "Will I go up and sort it out?" I'm conscious of being tired and also worried I won't be able to sort it. Also conscious at being pissed off having to drive so far. I do though, and get to a building, dank and dingy, a bit like the prison in *Midnight Express*. I see Donald through the crowd of bodies lying there on the stone floor. He gets up, says "thanks for coming, you've got to get me out". I say, "why are you here?" He is babbling and I can't make sense, I keep trying to get him to slow down. The other "prisoners" are in sackcloth and all lying huddled up together. Two black guys look up from the floor, tell us to shut up and start throwing things at us.' So that was one heavy night.

Here is another one, more pleasant, just as easy to work out. 'Looking at a picture of my Dad from a few years ago, when he was ill, and into the foreground came his face of about forty years ago, so that gradually the photo of him as an old man was replaced by the younger one. It was like a photo but his features were moving. Warm smile. He didn't say anything but I was pleased to see him. Felt real.'

If my dreams were indexed, Fiona would have the largest entry. On the political front, Tony is in there a fair bit, often fighting with Gordon, but also John Prescott features regularly, sometimes in a situation where he and I are arguing, in others where we are trying to sort out a problem for someone else. I seem to be in the north a lot, and I am at sporting events in my dreams just as often as in real life. And I am often getting lost, failing, or fearing failure as in this one, which followed my going to New Zealand as an advisor to the British and Irish Lions rugby team. 'I was at the last minute asked to play on the wing at a big game at Gloucester. I was very nervous, didn't think I was up to it. I contacted Mum, Dad and Donald and got them to come and watch. We went by coach to the ground. We put down our stuff in a crowded, dingy dressing room, got changed and out to warm up on a really bad pitch. Brown rather than green; dusty, bumpy. We did a series of warm-up exercises, then back in for the team talk, and back out to play. The first time the ball came to me, I was clattered to the ground and really hurt my shoulder. The physio came on. He asked if it was dislocated. I said I didn't know but it was agony. I couldn't move it. He said I would have to go off. I went off and into the empty dressing room. I was relieved but also a bit ashamed. I had a shower but the water was either too hot or cold, and there was no shampoo or soap. I found Donald in the bar and he was deep in conversation with someone who was moaning that I had been picked ahead of a local nineteen-year-old. As we left the bar the guy said "don't bother coming back". Then in a car to London with a couple of people asking me what I felt about the whole experience. I said I was pissed off. The coaches felt they had to pick me ahead of others who were more suited because they think I'm a big fish. But I'd have been happy to stay on the sidelines. And it means the press will have another field day saying I should have stayed out of rugby, never gone on the Lions tour, etc. I felt I'd let people down.'

My Best/Worst Log

In addition to my daily dream register, for months David made me write down every day my 'best/worst log', the best and the worst things that had happened on a given day. Sometimes it felt like a waste of time. But then he or I or both of us might see patterns that could become helpful. Both the dreams and the best/

worst log, certainly, showed up intense love for, and real anxiety about, the children, and a deep sense of conflict about my role in politics.

All very obvious, you might say. Who doesn't worry about their kids? Who wouldn't worry about the kind of political issues I was involved in? But two things were helpful. One was the way that a small detail might trigger a helpful insight, his or mine, when we discussed it. The second was that it helped me understand that I needed both my family life and my professional life, but I had to get them in better balance. David also felt my dreams revealed a 'propensity to beat yourself up too much', and he felt our analysis had helped me do less of that.

The sheer number of my dreams, and their intensity and sometimes violence, in which I was literally trapped, or immobile, or drowning, or incapacitated in some way, helped me to the realisation that no matter how big a sense of duty I felt to others, I also needed freedom, and release. I don't remember the specific discussions with David about any of them. I just know those discussions helped me to the insight that I must keep my freedom. I cannot be trapped.

Perhaps the reason Fiona and Tony figured most in my dreams at that time was because of the resentment I felt towards both for the pressures they put me under. But Fiona's resentment towards me, David believed, was more justified than the demands Tony put on me, especially after I 'left'.

'Women understand that sometimes men run off with another woman. If you did that, Fiona would not appreciate it, she would not be happy about it, but she would understand. It is what men have done forever. But she sees you running off not with another woman, but with a job, and she can't understand it, because she knows you know it damages you.'

That also helped me reframe the prism through which I looked at home and work. I didn't stop working, and never will. I didn't stop taking Tony's calls. But I didn't go running in response the way I once felt I had to. I at least thought about the impact on me, and on others, especially the family. Understanding (or at least looking at) my dreams did that, or helped to.

When things were bad with Fiona, David told me to do something for her I had never done before. So if I went out for a run, I might come home carrying a bunch of flowers as I ran back over Hampstead Heath, enjoying the smiles of those who saw me. Or arrange a trip to a place she had talked of wanting to see but had never been to. 'Isn't this just a bit of amateur marriage guidance?' I once protested.

'Less of the amateur,' replied the would-be saviour of the TBGBs.

This was about breaking patterns of behaviour, and the best/worst exercise was a way of seeing what the patterns were. 'For example,' he explained, 'the best times can be when someone is interacting with other people, and the worst when they are alone, or having to do something with others they would really rather not.

Freedom and entrapment are common themes in the best/worst scenario. But when people have identified what the issues are they often feel empowered to change them.'

Similarly, he said that asking patients to do something new, something they have never tried before, is about testing people's ability to change. If we are talking about trying to change the way we feel, showing that it is possible to change our own habits and patterns of behaviour is of itself a useful thing. Conversely, an inability to do so may indicate how badly we are trapped in our own damaging behaviours. 'This is a very good indication of someone's ability to change,' he explains. 'I'm astonished at how often people can't think of anything different or new to do. They prefer to "Stick with what you know!"'

So let me share with you some of the other exercises we did together, in the hope you might benefit from trying some of them for yourself.

Mindfulness

You may recall that when I asked David what was the point of life, he said the point was to live it. Similarly, he describes the role and purpose of mindfulness. 'It is all to do with staying in the moment, because that is what being alive is all about. We tend to fret about the past – but that's water under the bridge and has gone, we cannot press "undo". Or we worry about the future, which hasn't arrived. But while we're doing these things we're not in the moment, which is all we have. So mindfulness trains you to live in the moment, with everything that moment has to offer, its sights, smells, feelings, sensations; these will move on to other things so it's a bit like watching clouds go by but paying full attention to them while they're there. Then focusing on the next "cloud" that comes into view. It's a peaceful and relaxing form of meditation and seems very helpful in alleviating stress and anxiety.'

I have never found this easy. That is because I do 'fret', to use his word, about the past and, even more so, I ruminate excessively about the future, often imagining the worst, catastrophising. Even if, as often happens, I can feel myself absorbed in nice music or wonderful scenery, I struggle to hold my mind in place sufficiently for me to stay in the moment rather than stray back to the past or forward to the future.

So when David asked me to spend time doing nothing more than looking at a raisin in my hand, and seeing where my thoughts took me, I agreed to do so with little expectation that it would do any good. That it did may have been as much about external circumstances at the time, but for whatever reason, I found myself drawn into a detailed, concentrated study of the raisin. He said it was important just to let it happen, to persevere, even if it felt a bit weird at first – comical even; it did, as I asked myself, 'why the fuck am I sitting here staring at a raisin?'. Keep rolling it around your hand and you will start to see it in different ways. I did.

I started to see just how complicated it was, with its lines and shades and contours. How different it looked from this one rather than that one. How the little curves and cracks would move as if they had a little life of their own. Then suddenly my thoughts were going nowhere. They were just there, and there was nothing in the world I was thinking of, other than this soft, gnarled raisin. There was a beauty and a meaning in there, and for the first time I began to see what David was getting at.

Gratitude Versus Resentment

He asked me to write a gratitude list, and a resentment list, and 'see which comes out longer'. When I asked why, as ever he had a simple explanation. 'Resentments', he said, 'fuel addictive behaviours and help to keep people sick.' So we find ourselves giving reasons to ourselves to justify damaging behaviour, and to continue with it.

Rather than ditch resentments, we hang onto them, to provide the justification. 'If you had my life, you'd drink too.' Most people can find something they consider to be an unfairness or sadness in their lives, resentment at which can be used in this way. It means, says David, that 'resentments can become a focus in people's lives'.

Drawing up a gratitude list, he says, is a way of finding the flip side of that coin. 'There are so many things in life we can be grateful for but which we often take for granted,' he says. 'Having food and shelter, companionship, a helping hand, the person who noticed you and said "good morning" – these are all to do with being in the world and a part of it. Loving parents, kids who care, being able to ask for what we need and often getting it.' Forcing yourself to think about and genuinely appreciate these things we take for granted is a way of taking stock, of seeing that despite how we feel, we may have more to be thankful for than angry about. Here are my gratitude and resentment lists, for instance.

Gratitude List

Three children growing up mainly happy, healthy and well.

Grateful for their love, humour, ambitions and enthusiasms, and for their ability to lift me and give me more happiness than anyone or anything else.

A partner who has stayed with me in an enduring relationship when many others might not have.

Fiona's love and support (most of the time).

Her practical sustenance of me and the kids.

Her amazing organisational and home-building skills.

The fact I don't have to worry about money and practicalities because she takes care of it all.

A sister always there for me as I am for her.

An extended family challenging yet supportive.

A mother-in-law adored by all.

Fond memories of father, mother and father-in-law, and a sense of their spirit and guidance in us.

The dog.

Genuine friends.

Strong memories of absent friends.

Good holidays in a place the family all love.

The ability to make the kids laugh.

The ability to make most people laugh.

The ability to enjoy laughter.

The ability to connect with most people.

The knowledge I can give the kids a lot of what they want.

A nice home with good neighbours.

Demonic energy when not depressed.

The ability, most of the time, to sleep easily at night.

Hampstead Heath.

Regent's Park Canal.

Having been born in a good country to live in (pre-Brexit shit-show).

Scottish heritage.

The ability to play the bagpipes.

The ability to speak foreign languages.

Reasonable health.

Low resting pulse rate.

Fitness to run long distances, often in beautiful places.

Connection with charities that help me do good
and take part in interesting events.

Never having to fear hunger.

The ability to write.

Knowing I have a platform for anything I want to
say.

Being articulate.

Being in demand.

Having beliefs I hold strongly.

Knowing many interesting people around the
world.

A love of sport.

Burnley Football Club. The fans, the passion, the
friendships.

The fact Calum supports them too.

My Pinarello bike.

Working in sport.

Having been a personal friend of the PM and
others in government, and still trusted to be
confided in and have advice sought.

Extraordinary experiences and memories of a
political life.

Having had the opportunity to build and lead
teams.

Having seen the world.

Knowing personally Bush, Clinton, Putin, Chirac,
Mandela et al.

Being able to say – every day – I played with
Maradona and Pele!

Having a ridiculous contacts book.

A reputation for being good at what I do.
Many offers of new opportunities.
The ability to say no to most of them.
A love of so much music, and so many books.
Jacques Brel.
Elvis.
Edith Piaf.
France Gall.
Motown.
Diana Ross.
Frankie Valli.
Northern Soul.
Abba.
Being tall.
Courage.
The ability to appreciate simple things – a glass of
    water, a walk, a run.
An appreciation of great scenery.
Dreams.

Resentment List

Asthma.
Depression.
Feeling I ought to get more sustained happiness
    than I do.
Feeling misunderstood despite supposedly being
    a good communicator.
My inability to make bad situations in my own
    life better, when I can do it for others.

Feeling that Fiona has the same inability when it
comes to me.

In part, resenting my reputation, though I also
know it is what sets me apart.

Resentment bordering on hatred of much of the
media, its herd instinct, its self-importance and
its corrosive impact upon political debate. The
superficiality of most commentators.

Crap TV.

Celebrity magazines.

Drugs and their impact.

Cynicism about politics being thought to be trendy.

Litter – and therefore the people responsible.

Being smoked upon.

People who can't be bothered to vote.

Self-indulgent MPs who care more about their
vanity than maintaining a Labour government.

Patients who miss NHS appointments.

Parents who don't control their kids, or check
their bad behaviour.

Parents who don't support teachers.

Not being clear re future.

Feeling I was forced to do something I didn't
want to (leave job).

Sales phone calls.

Private education.

Snobbery.

Racism.

Misogyny.

Polluting cars.

Dog owners who don't clear up after them on the
   Heath.
People thinking they're being original when
   saying something you've often heard before.
Chewing gum.
Ketchup.
Eating in cinemas.
Bad service in restaurants.

Definitely time to stop – I'm beginning to sound like a
bloody taxi driver. Gratitude wins, easily – I just need
to be grateful for it.

The Need–Want Exercise

Write down a list of statements beginning with the
words 'I want' and another list beginning with 'I need'.

The thinking behind this one is similar to the gratitude versus resentment exercise. It is also a way of forcing ourselves to think clearly about the difference
between needing and wanting. 'We often mix up the
two,' says David. 'What we need may not be what we
want – for example, we might need to be taken to
account over certain aspects of our life but we may not
want to be. Or we may want to have recognition for
something we've done but we may not need to have it.
That shouldn't stop us from doing it again.'

Here is my list.

I want to be happy.

I want to stay with Fiona and our relationship to
  be strong.

I want the kids to be happy and fulfilled.

I want them to stay in touch when they move
  away.

I want to make a difference.

I want to be able to decide my future.

I want to do another marathon faster than the last
  one.

I want to enjoy holidays.

I want to do interesting things.

I want a new challenge, but not yet.

I need my family.

I need the children to be happy and fulfilled.

I need to work.

I need to make a difference.

I need to be validated by Fiona especially.

I need to be stimulated.

I need a new challenge.

I need to stop drinking again.

I need to keep fit.

I need big moments.

The Other Side of the Coin

One of his exercises reminded me of when my Hutton
Inquiry lawyer, Jonathan Sumption QC, described the

law as 'public relations with a wig on'. I suggested to David that psychiatry was 'spin with a white coat on' after he asked me to write down everything that irritated me about Fiona, and turn it into a positive statement. (But, annoyingly enough, it works.)

She shouts too much . . . she is good at keeping order.

She talks too loudly to the cleaner . . . very clear in instructions. House-proud.

Constantly going over bad things in the past . . . why shouldn't she? Most were caused by me. Learn from them.

Self-pity at being taken for granted . . . don't take her for granted then, you Muppet.

Spendthrift . . . really makes the house look nice. Dresses beautifully. Buys great presents.

Always gets the expensive option . . . believes in quality.

And so on, like that.

Then there are the times he has asked me to write about a particular theme or issue, taking those we have discussed and getting me to think about them more between sessions, so that the thinking is honed.

As, for instance, the following:

Humility

'We are all important to ourselves and to others around us. But in the grand sweep of history, and amid the grand force of nature, we are but grains of sand. We seek to control the world around us as best we can, to bring order to what otherwise might be chaos, and we may have some limited success. But there are forces bigger than all of us. History. Time. Nature. We can shape history. But we cannot stop time. We can mow the lawn and prune flowers, but it is other forces that make them grow.

We can leave but a small stamp on the world. The morning after we die, some will mourn, but most will carry on unaware. It will be the same when they go. The world carries on turning. Airports carry on shipping people around the world from one soulless conveyor belt to another.

There are points in our life when we feel we matter more than others. When we feel stronger than others, when we feel we own our own universe. But at any point in our life, had I died, had you died, the world would have gone on. There is no job on earth that cannot be filled by others tomorrow.

In our workplaces, in our countries, it sometimes feels like there are big people and there are little people. The big people are bosses. They have power and authority. I was a big person. But the big people can't function without the little people. The little people can't always do the big people's job, but often the big people can't do the little people's job. The Prime Minister could not get to his meeting with the President without drivers, pilots, security staff, secretaries, typists, translators and so on. They are all part of a team. If one part doesn't function properly, the whole doesn't function properly. My basic belief is that we are all of equal worth. Not that we are all the same, or capable of being the same, or desirous of being the same, but that we are all human beings who owe our existence to others and who cannot function without others. We are all of equal worth.

I always respected the driver, the cleaner, the messenger every bit as much as the big people. I never spoke down to those below me in a work structure, and I regularly challenged those above me, often on behalf of those supposedly below me.

A blade of grass has as complex a life as we do. It is part of what we are. Trees can outlive us. There are animals which lack our brainpower, but exceed us in terms of courage and might.

Fear can humble. It makes us confront our limits and our mortality.

Anger can humble. It diminishes us.

Emotion can humble. I get moved to tears by sporting success. By national anthems sung at the Olympics. By crowds at football matches where one club survives and another goes down.

Change can humble, for we can be reminded of past failings.

We can learn humility if we learn from mistakes.

Great art and music can humble for it is the work of minds more creative than ours.

Poverty can humble because it sees people tolerate a life we cannot contemplate.

The process of life is humbling. The human body is humbling. The human mind is humbling.

There but for the grace of God. We could all be the down-and-out, the vagrant, the battered wife, the abused child, the man with the dead-end job, the prostitute enslaved. Be thankful we are not, spare a thought for those who are, do what we can to help them. We are our brother's keeper.

Great buildings and other creations. Bridges. Tunnels. How the hell do they make them? Think how many little people and big people were involved.

We must not be so humble as to ignore our strength, or fail to use it . . .

"The only thing necessary for the triumph of evil is for good men to do nothing."' (Edmund Burke)

There is just one exercise I have so far refused to do, despite David trying for years to get me to. It has become known to me, him and to Fiona as 'the croft plan'. It is that I should go and live in a croft, on my own, with supplies for at least a month, no communications with the outside world, no calls in or out (though we would have a system for emergencies), no help with cooking, cleaning or catering, no TV, no radio. Books allowed. Writing most definitely allowed. Long walks allowed but no contact to be made with others. He is obsessed with the idea, and swears that others who have done it now swear by it too. But why, I ask? What will happen? The truth, he says, will bubble up.

'But I have told you the truth.'

'Yes, I am sure you have, but you still get depressed, and we still don't know why. This would really strip things down. For someone who is *so* connected with people, places and things in the *outside* world, being deprived of that and having more of your *inside* world can be beneficial and revealing. I know I've told you that you should never go into your own head unaccompanied but I think the croft situation would be OK. You would be facing your fear and finding out what that's all about.'

I sometimes think David feels there is some deep hidden secret in my childhood that we have never dug out of my subconscious, and if only I would let it be dug out I would have the key to understanding myself. Fiona tends to agree, finding it odd that I have so few actual memories of my childhood. But I really don't think there is. I have a bad memory, full stop. It is partly why I keep a diary. My parents were good parents, if obviously from different backgrounds to the one in which they raised me, and they were also old-fashioned, by their generation and in their attitudes. But my mother was always there for us, she saw that as her role, and though my Dad could be strict he was certainly never cruel, often very kind, always supportive in matters to do with interests, sport, education, career.

So why am I so resistant to the idea of a month or two all on my own? Partly, I am not sure I could cope, practically. I have never cooked. I cannot change a plug. I hate to admit it but when it comes to practicalities, I am the pits. I am also – for all that I like silence at times, and only like crowds at sporting events or (some) political rallies, and hate most parties – quite sociable, and I would miss people, especially family and close friends. So I am resisting, and have for years. But he keeps trying, and I suspect he will until I cave in. We shall see.

Perhaps I am also resistant because I am actually, despite the plunges, so much better and happier than I was. It is why I dedicated *All in the Mind* to him and Dr Bennie. They were important strokes of luck in my life, and my route from madness to something more akin to fulfilment. Psychiatry and especially these two psychiatrists have had a big impact on my life, for the better.

14

TO MEDICATE OR
NOT TO MEDICATE

It is strange that I, who never took illegal drugs at university, who can still feel my gorge rising when Grace casually talks about drugs she has taken, should now so heavily rely on antidepressants. Fiona has always felt David is too 'trigger happy' with the medication he prescribes me. Her face was a real picture when I told her he wanted me to take the anti-epilepsy drug. It is fair to say I have had as many misses as hits. I can't even remember all their names any more, or what they did – escitalopram, duloxetine, venlafaxine, mirtazapine, all ring a bell. But there was one that made me so tired I couldn't stay awake in meetings and so wired I couldn't sleep at night. I knocked that on the head pretty smartish.

I was always keen to come off medication anyway. Back to wanting to solve it all myself. But finally, after a decade or so, we seem to have found the one that works. I think sertraline is my new addiction.

'Am I going to be on this forever?' I ask.

'I don't know. It's up to you.'

'No. It's up to you.'

'Do you want to come off it?'

'Well I'd rather not be on it.'

'Is it making you feel better?'

'Yes.'

'So why do you want to come off it?'

Pause.

'I just do.'

'Do you remember the last time you came off it?'

'No.'

'You crashed a month later.'

'Did I?'

'Yes. Badly.'

'Oh.'

'If you find something that helps you live life, Alastair, let it help you.'

But it is possible that if I had met Joanna Moncrieff before I met David, I would never have known what sertraline was, let alone allowed it to become a fixture in my morning ritual, which starts with what I call my three 'S's – shave, sertraline, symbicort (asthma drug), brush teeth, start day.

Joanna Moncrieff is a founding member of the Critical Psychiatry Network, formed of psychiatrists around the world who reject the idea that mental illness can or should be viewed in the same way as physical illness. They fear the medical profession is in the grip of the pharmaceutical industry, that doctors dole out anti-depressants far too easily and that there are other and better ways to treat depression. The titles of her books, *The Myth of the Chemical Cure* and *The Bitterest Pill*, give you a sense of where she is coming from.

'The problem is they alter the way the mind works,' she told me, as we went for a stroll in Regent's Park on a cold, crisp morning.

'But that is why I take them. I *want* my mind to alter when it feels like shit.'

'Yes, but the pills don't just change the bad bits. They're mind-altering substances in the sense that they alter normal mental functions and emotions, not just ones that are pathological or unwanted. There's this idea that we're giving drugs to tweak the bad bits, tweak the bits of your mental functioning that are not working properly or the bits you don't like, but it's not like that. They're much cruder than that, and they're altering mental functions in a general way. We're viewing it in the wrong way, we're treating it as if it were a disease the same as diabetes or cancer, when actually, it's a different sort of thing and it needs a different sort of response. Just encouraging people to go to their GP and get medication is really not the answer.'

Physical illness, she insists, is totally different. 'There is such a thing as diabetes that we can look at and investigate and research independently from the people who have it. Depression is not like that. It's always connected to the individual who has it and you can't really deal with it in the abstract. So the problem when we're doling out antidepressants is that we might be encouraging people to see themselves as having a lifelong, underlying weakness, rather than something that they might be able to get to grips with and manage in the long term. I think sometimes medication can say to people, "you know, I'm weak, I'm vulnerable, I've got this condition". So what are you going to do? Have it forever?'

Her scepticism about antidepressants developed very early in her career, after she graduated from Newcastle University in 1989. 'I was prescribing antidepressants as a junior doctor, but I couldn't convince myself that they really made much difference. Some people got better; some people didn't. It didn't seem to be greatly related to whether they had an antidepressant or not. There seemed to be other things that would predict whether they got better or not.' Those who saw their condition improve, she felt, did so because the key relationships in their life improved, or a burden that had been weighing them down was lifted, or they simply thought through the problems that had been making them ill, and found a way to understand and address them better. 'And then, of course, there were lots of people who didn't get better at all. They tried one antidepressant and then another antidepressant and then another one, and they didn't seem to make much difference.'

She started to study the placebo control trials, and it confirmed her view that doctors were rushing too quickly to the prescription pad, not least because they didn't have the time to go through all the underlying issues, such as work and home circumstances, that might have brought the patient through the surgery door. 'It's about trying to identify the problems that each individual has, and trying to work out ways that they can be tackled. And sometimes a psychiatrist might be able to help people think through those difficulties. Therapy can do that better than medication, I think.'

The drug companies, though we all need the drugs they make, and more so as we age, have never exactly had a positive profile, despite the evident good their products do. Thalidomide casts a long shadow, as do the now largely outlawed marketing practices designed to capture the medical professions. But Dr Moncrieff believes that I and millions like me, and our doctors, are indeed victims of such a pharma-capture, related to serotonin, a natural chemical produced both in the gut and, to a lesser extent, in the brain.

'It's thought that there's an association between low serotonin levels in the brain and depression,' she explains, 'and therefore, having more serotonin circulating around might alleviate the depression. My problem with this is that there really isn't any evidence that low serotonin causes depression or is even associated with it. This was promoted by pharmaceutical companies back in the 1990s when they had this new set of drugs that affected serotonin and they marketed them alongside the idea that depression was a chemical imbalance, and specifically a serotonin imbalance. It was a myth. It just became very widely accepted and wasn't questioned and still isn't really questioned now. But if you try and pin anyone down on it, they can't really come up with any convincing evidence that shows it.'

'But how do you explain that since taking the pills I am on, though yes I do still get depressed, I have felt better?'

'I can ask you – how do you know it is the pills that have done that? If you just take one individual, it's always difficult to know whether it's the antidepressant or whether you've come to terms better with your problems, are better at dealing with them, better at dealing with your emotions?'

'But they do change the brain, you said that earlier.'

'Yes, they are not inert, they're not placebo tablets, they do change the brain. We haven't really investigated very thoroughly what sort of changes they produce. They are quite subtle brain-changing tablets. Sertraline is an SSRI, a selective serotonin reuptake inhibitor. There are some studies that show that some people report side effects such as an emotional blunting, feeling a bit lethargic sometimes.'

'I have had that with other drugs,' I counter, 'but not this one.'

'But have you made other changes in your life that might have contributed to you feeling better?'

And, of course, I have. I used to see sleep as a waste of time, hours lost from the pursuit of progress, or pleasure, and the alleviation of boredom, which has always been one of my driving fears. Earlier I mentioned young reporter Geordie Greig, now editor of the *Daily Mail*. I remember when I was his news editor, heading for a breakdown, telling him he should train himself to get by with three or four hours' sleep. Always a diplomat, he smiled and nodded, pretending to take me seriously. Now I am obsessed with sleeping long, and well. A night in bed before ten p.m., and sod watching the news, is a night well spent. My diet, not least thanks to Fiona being a health freak and a good cook, is vastly improved. I exercise pretty much every day. 'Read books not newspapers' is a relatively new motto, which has definitely helped my mental health. 'Listen to music not the *Today* programme, or learn to enjoy silence.' All good, all good.

I have got a much better balance between my love of my family and my continuing workaholic tendencies, although I am writing this book on what is meant to be our annual summer holiday in France. I have already interrupted it to travel to Australia to speak about and campaign on mental health, on which I have written and published several long reads; to write and do media on my decision no longer to try to stay in the Labour Party; to take part in regular conference calls on the People's Vote campaign; to prepare for a series of events at the Edinburgh Festival; and this afternoon I hope to ride my bike up Mont Ventoux. 'This is not', I can hear David Sturgeon saying through a smile, 'how normal people behave on holiday.' Fair point, but I am enjoying myself, I am spending a lot of time with Fiona and the children, and the balance is better than it used to be. Rory arrives with his girlfriend today. Calum has just been with us for ten days. Grace is making her debut at the Edinburgh Fringe and we speak several times a day. I am having a holiday my way, honest.

Dr Moncrieff thinks age might have played a part in my seeming recovery. 'I think we do get better at managing our emotions as we get older, don't we? We know ourselves better.'

'But why do I still get depression?' It is a question I ask of every psychiatrist I meet, and they rarely give the same answer. 'I have dug away, and dug away, and I just don't know. It just comes on me,' I said.

'It is not easy to pinpoint what it is,' she replies. 'Sometimes I think depression is exactly that – it is a signal; it is a signal to you to look at your life and see what it is that might be wrong. We've given people the wrong message, that depression is a chemical thing, whereas maybe it's a lot more complicated than that.'

She picked up on something I had said earlier, half in jest – that I worried sertraline was my latest addiction, the latest toy for my addictive personality to play with. When I once made the same crack with David, he became, rarely for him, a little defensive, saying simply: 'They are not drugs of addiction, not addictive in themselves.'

Dr Moncrieff's response was very different. 'There is such a thing as psychological addiction. People feel they need them when maybe they don't. Because, of course, if you take antidepressants at a time when you're feeling very low and then you start feeling better, even if it's nothing to do with the antidepressants, you're going to think it is, and probably be quite frightened at the idea of stopping them.'

'*Quite frightened at the idea of stopping them . . .*' That resonated with me, loudly. The fear is partly born, as David has reminded me many times, of the huge plunges that have tended to follow my coming off medication before.

'That is absolutely where I am, because before, I've always agitated to get off them, and if I've been feeling reasonably OK, I've tapered down slowly, then off completely, and a massive plunge has usually followed, sometimes in days, sometimes weeks, but it always came. Whereas this time I've stayed on this one for three years, and though I have still got depressed, I've definitely felt better.'

'I normally say to people who are in that situation that it's probably best to continue, and there may come a time when you feel you are over it, you're totally confident, and then you might be able to stop. But while you're not feeling that, while you're still feeling that you may be vulnerable, it's probably best you carry on. I suppose what worries me is that if you think that you've got better because of the antidepressants, you may actually underrate what you have done to help yourself get better. You may not be giving yourself enough credit or recognising that the other things you're doing have been helpful.'

When I left Dr Moncrieff I was in a state of some confusion. She is, like David, a trained psychiatrist. She has enormous empathy and wisdom, and a humanity that shines out of her, just as it shines out of him. Yet her views are so different to his. And of course David admits that whenever he is prescribing drugs, or asking me to 'do your homework' through all the exercises he sets me, he does not know for sure what will or won't work. 'Trial and error.' Trial and error has taken me to sertraline, and we both feel it works. But Dr Moncrieff thinks it is a happy coincidence, and that the continuing use of a mind-altering drug could be doing more harm than good. When we think about science, we like to think, well, that means there's a problem and science is giving you a solution. But when it comes to mental illness, so much of it is about opinion.

When I was struggling with alcohol, after I stopped drinking I became conscious of the fact we all, whether we drink or not, have a 'relationship' with drink. Likewise we have a relationship with our mental health, and in some ways sertraline has become like the guidance counsellor in my relationship with my depression. It seems to help, and while it seems to help, I think it would be crazy of me to come off it. I'd love to think I'd never get depression again, that some day fairly soon I'll come off the antidepressants and never go back on them. I'd love to think that. Right now, I think it's a bit unrealistic.

This is why I admire the best psychiatrists. They don't have X-rays to look at. All they have to go on is what they see, and what they hear, when the patient is in front of them; and given so many of their patients struggle to communicate when depressed, they have to dig and dig and dig until they mine something useful. But even then, they don't, as David has often admitted to me, know for certain what will or won't happen.

So we are left with trust, and I trust him. I could easily have grown to trust Dr Moncrieff. But I got to David first. For now, I am staying put, albeit that I reflect on what she said most mornings, as the pill goes down once more.

15

CLASS A DRUGS

Having never smoked cannabis, let alone taken anything stronger on the illegal drugs front, I couldn't quite believe where I was heading on the next step of my exploration, and nor could Grace, who finds my obsessive anti-drugs outlook as comical as it is antediluvian. The idea that I was on my way to check out whether a Class A drug based on the ingredients of magic mushrooms might help me had her in hysterics. I fear I have given Grace a fruitful new strand for her next stand-up show, as she starts to mimic what I would be like high on drugs.

The magic mushrooms drug is called psilocybin, and to see whether it might be worth my trying, I meet Ian Roullier – who has taken it as part of an experiment involving patients who have been resistant to anti-depressants – and the woman who ran the trials, Dr Ros Watts, clinical psychologist at the Psychedelic Research Group at Imperial College London.

I think depressives often have a sixth sense about other depressives. As we sit in the upstairs room of a café in Islington, North London, there is something in Ian's eyes that gives it away. He definitely has it.

Ian endured horrific abuse at the hands of his father. 'It's an awful thing to say, I know, but I hope his death is slow and painful. He's out there in the real world again, now, without a care in the world. But what he actually did, I mean, how do you move on from that? How do you get beyond it? It's a really tough one. So, I can't really let go of that and I can't let go of the feeling "I hope you die soon and I hope you die a slow, painful death". Awful as it is to say that, on a whole compassion level for everyone, I can't extend that to him.'

Ian has been at nine on my depression scale, and tempted by ten, many times. Within minutes of meeting, we were sharing stories of how we have imagined our deaths, and rationalised suicidal feelings by persuading ourselves it would be good for our loved ones.

He shares my anger when people speak of suicide as 'selfish'.

He said he thought of taking his own life purely 'to stop my wife suffering'.

'It's like you are really trying to save those around you and you just want to stop all the suffering. You want them to stop suffering and you want to stop suffering yourself. And it seems like the only way to do that, the logical way to do that, is to do away with yourself, to kill yourself.'

Whereas my depressions tend to start as a cloud above me, he says his strike as 'this feeling in the solar plexus, a knot, a dark, horrible weight that can really intensify. And if the pressure builds up to such a great extent there would be angry outbursts, verbally. I'd throw my phone across the room, or push a wardrobe into a window. And then you have the self-recrimination, and the guilt. I remember after one outburst, I sat upstairs for a couple of hours with my head in my hands and got to a point where I felt that to prevent myself from harming those closest to me it would be best if I wasn't there any more. It felt logical rather than instinctive. It felt like the right thing for me to do for those around me to save them, stop the pain for them.'

Thankfully Ian's wife has both empathy and humour, and when he talked her through his plan to end it all as an act of love for her as much as to end the pain for himself, she said: 'If you do that, I'll kill you.'

'It may sound dramatic, but I think without her, I wouldn't be here now. I'd be long gone.'

He has had chronic depression for most of his life, been in and out of hospital, on and off different forms of medication, but nothing much seemed to work.

Together, the three of us watch a video taken of Ian as he was given the drug in two separate sessions in the trial being run by Dr Watts. He is given ten milligrams for the first, twenty-five milligrams for the second a week later.

MEDIC: How are you feeling now?
IAN: There's apprehension, but there's also excitement as well, and it feels like an adventure. Letting go is difficult for me. I feel a bit scared.

MEDIC: Why don't you try it and then come back
   to us and tell us what you experience?
IAN: It's really intense. I'm really scared of losing
   control. Scared I'll go mad. Scared I'll die.

When at one point Ian started to laugh, I stopped
the film to ask him why. 'It was the Wizard of Oz
moment,' he said. 'It was like I pulled back the
curtain and there he [his father] was and he wasn't
Superman, he was just a silly little man who couldn't
harm me any more.' Other times, though, he was
clearly reliving the worst of the feelings engendered
by the abuse, and it was disturbing to watch, even
more so switching my gaze from the film to Ian's
reaction to it in real time.

The good news was that after his two sessions, he
had several months free of depression and anxiety – a
long time for him. The bad news was that the licence
allowing Ros Watts and her team to administer the drug
was time-limited for the period of the research
programme, and for him to keep taking the drugs now
would be to break the law. Their disappointment was
palpable. 'I'm back on antidepressants and anti-anxiety
medication. I feel disconnected again. I don't fully feel
sometimes that I'm really participating in life. The
psilocybin helped me a lot, but it's not a miracle cure,
so here I am back on sertraline and pregabalin.'

Of the twenty people on the trial, three didn't
respond to the drug at all, either for better or worse.
Eleven people had the same response as Ian: a few

months of remission from depression, with either no symptoms at all or very mild ones compared with what they were used to, and then the depression started to come back again. Six people, in the round of interviews six months after the experiment, had remained free of depression. Some of those have since relapsed, but two remain free of any depression from the treatment after two years. One of them described the effect of taking psilocybin as 'like turning on the lights in a dark house, and then the lights gradually faded again but I could never forget what I'd seen when the lights were on'.

Dr Watts describes the effects as the difference between an antibiotic and a painkiller. 'If you take a painkiller for a toothache, it numbs the pain but it doesn't do anything about the infection. So if you take an antibiotic, it heals the infection. Antidepressants are the painkiller, this is the antibiotic.' Ian concurs. 'Antidepressants for me are a way of dealing with the symptoms. They help you cope day to day, and that's extremely valuable in itself. Whereas psilocybin was really about dealing with the root causes and delving really deeply, feeling all of these things that you've hidden away for so long.' This, Dr Watts believes, explains the success. 'It uncovers unconscious material that they haven't been thinking about.'

I found Ian and his story profoundly moving. In the few hours we had together I could get a sense of his character, the damage done to him by the persistent abuse, and also the many ups and downs of his life since. And while I am neither scientist nor medic, I could see just how deeply he felt he had benefited from the experience, how much he had gained from those few months free of depression, and how much he and Dr Watts wished he could have another go, and see if it worked as well, or even better, second time around. 'It is very frustrating,' she said.

The experience has led me on another step towards a different way of thinking about drugs. I was heading in that direction anyway, after reading *Chasing the Scream*, where journalist Johann Hari spent time with people involved in every aspect of the drugs trade, and reached the convincing conclusion that the so-called war on drugs was failing, and a new approach was required. I have been moving towards some form of decriminalisation, and certainly greater access for possible medical benefits, ever since. Hari has also written a superb book on depression, where like me he is keen to find new ways of dealing with it.

I found myself certain that Ian should be allowed to take more of this Class A drug, genuinely sorry and more than a little angry that he can't. To say I was surprised at my reaction is putting it mildly. It's a fundamental change in attitude for someone like me, with the passionately anti-drug views I have had most of my life, not least at Cambridge where I saw it as my mission to duff up posh-boy dealers. If Dr Watts had walked through my front door the day after my self-harming incident on Hampstead Heath and said, 'listen, we've got this trial we're doing, here is what it is, why don't you try it, you have nothing to lose', I reckon I would have done it.

16

ELECTRIC SHOCK

When Donald was in the military psychiatric hospital in Netley, after a while I became sufficiently part of the daytime furniture to wander around the place without staff wondering who I was or what I was up to. Most of them knew I was the brother of Donald the Scots Guards piper, and if I was mooching around on my own, it probably meant Donald was sleeping, or seeing one of the medics.

On one of these wanderings, I was walking along a corridor with offices to my left and, to my right, a kind of mezzanine, which overlooked a row of medical examination rooms below. When I looked down, I found myself watching one of the patients being administered what I later learned to be electroconvulsive therapy (ECT). A patient had electrodes applied to each temple, and a doctor was operating a machine at the far end of the bed. It was not as dramatic as the scenes in *One Flew Over the Cuckoo's Nest*, but certainly there was something deeply shocking about the sight of the man's body going into total spasm, when the convulsive moment came. The doctor looked up and spotted me, but my immediate instinct that I should walk on and pretend I had seen nothing faded when he smiled, as though to say he didn't object to my presence at all. Perhaps he thought I was a member of staff, I don't know, but certainly it felt like I was watching something I shouldn't.

I don't remember if this was before or after they had decided that Donald should have ECT treatment, and I asked if I could be with him when it was administered. They said I could, warning me I might find it upsetting. Donald was given an anaesthetic – I think general, certainly he was not awake during any of it – and perhaps that was what was so horrifying about the convulsion, which appeared something like an epileptic fit, while he was effectively asleep. As to whether the treatment was effective, I have no idea, but that was not the last time he had it, and Donald talked many times in later years about how he hated having ECT.

Not least because of *One Flew Over the Cuckoo's Nest*, and its role in popular culture and our understanding of severe mental illness, ECT has long had something of a bad reputation, though my own psychiatrist and many others argue it remains an effective treatment for several mental disorders, including persistent severe depression. I have since reflected that culture has played a significant role in cementing the stigma around mental illness. I don't blame Ken Kesey for writing such a novel, Miloš Forman for wanting to turn it into a film, or Jack Nicholson for giving such an intense performance. It was released in 1975, around the time Donald was coming to terms with having to leave the Army, and it remains a go-to cultural reference for mental illness even many years later. Go further back, to 1886, and I doubt that Robert Louis Stevenson would ever have imagined that his Gothic novella, *The Strange Case of Dr Jekyll and Mr Hyde*, would have entered the language in the way that it has, not least in the way we talk about people with schizophrenia as 'having a split personality – Jekyll and Hyde'.

I remembered one of Donald's psychiatrists telling me that one of the hardest parts of his work, when diagnosing a new patient with schizophrenia, was telling the family. 'You have to spend so much time telling them what it is not, rather than what it is, because of the way it is portrayed, the Jack Nicholson film, Jekyll and Hyde, and the press coverage of "psycho killers told by Jesus to murder". You will be amazed', he said, 'how many people think their son or daughter will end up in jail, because schizophrenia will drive them to kill someone.' In truth, the mentally ill are far more likely to be the victims of violence than its perpetrators.

I was not considered suitable for ECT, but for my next exploration I went to have what might be seen as a downscaled version of it, and this time I took Grace along with me. It is partly her desire for me to be off my daily dose of antidepressants that has led me to explore alternative approaches to treating depression. Of our three children, Grace has always been the one most enquiring about my depression, most in my face in demanding to know what is going on when my mood plunges and, most importantly, asking 'what should we do when it happens?' She was also not just very fond of Donald, but also fascinated by his illness.

Grace has had her own mental health issues, not least when she went to study French in Paris. One day, a few months into her course, she called me, and I could tell she wanted to come home, but didn't want to say so. 'Grace,' I said, 'if this is making you unhappy, just come home.' When she did come back, she saw someone – still does – to help deal with anxiety, switched from languages in Paris to film in London, and though she still struggles with anxiety from time to time, has never really looked back.

When we talked about my depression, she just wanted me to be happy all the time, in the way parents want their kids to be happy. She wanted me to be free of depression, and though she saw the pills helped, the fact that the depressions still came, albeit less often and in the main less intensely, meant to her that 'the drugs don't work'.

Grace was particularly fascinated that I was prepared to try this 'kind of mini-ECT', three letters which ever since witnessing Donald's treatment in Netley have held a mix of fear and horror for me. It involved going to the Institute of Cognitive Research, University College London, to meet Vince Walsh, Professor of Human Brain Research.

Professor Walsh first tested on my arm the magnetic field he was about to pass through my scalp as part of the TMS treatment he was about to administer. Not *Test Match Special* – something that is always good for mental wellbeing, except when Geoff Boycott strays into politics – but a Transcranial Magnetic Stimulator. The test on my arm did nothing more than reveal my squeamishness in the face of all matters medical, as the tiny electrical impulse had me jumping from my chair. Professor Walsh immediately identified the problem. 'Wimp,' he snorted.

Apparently my fear was to do with being a control freak. 'I knew that you'd be a nervous subject because you're not in control and you don't like that. That twitch is your anxiety, it's just you being nervous. There is no neurological reason to react like that at all.'

When he transferred me to a chair, applied a rather clunky contraption to my temple, and started the treatment, the feeling was as though a gentle woodpecker was pecking repeatedly at the side of my head. Neither pleasant nor painful. What was happening, he explained, was that he was able to direct the machine specifically to stimulate local parts of the brain – selectively excite some parts and temporarily deactivate others.

The idea behind TMS derives from ECT – the introduction of an electrical current into the brain – but TMS wasn't an attempt to make a machine that does what ECT does; its invention followed that of the machine. In any event, he argues that while ECT remains the most effective treatment for chronic depression, with 'a higher success rate than anything else', TMS can be administered without anaesthesia, without an epileptic seizure, without memory loss and with no side effects beyond a mild headache.

It is less of a huge shock to the whole system, more a direct hit on the parts that need to be hit. He explains that when I am depressed, there is under-activity in the frontal parts of the brain. This treatment is trying to increase the levels of serotonin in my brain.

'So, I am passing a large magnetic field through your scalp, it meets your brain tissue and that induces a magnetic field in your brain. But it's a small electrical field and very focal. ECT isn't very focal, you see it stimulating all over the head. With this, you can stimulate really restrictive regions of the brain.'

Antidepressants have a thirty per cent chance of success. 'So ask yourself, if I'm in my early episode of depression, do I take antidepressants that have a one in three chance of working, with side effects like weight gain, loss of sex drive, interfering with my sleep? Or should I have a go at this, which has none of those side effects, and none of the side effects associated with ECT either?'

With ECT, you know it is connecting when the patient goes into epileptic seizure. This is mild, almost pleasant, by comparison. 'There is no risk,' he says, 'and from around the world a lot of evidence of success. I would suggest it is more effective than any given anti-depressant – the jury is in on that. The question for me is why isn't it on every psychiatrist's treatment options.'

For people like me, perhaps his next sentence provided the answer. 'One of the things I like about introducing this to patients and to psychiatrists is that it's proactive, you have to decide to turn up for this every day, for half an hour, for four weeks, with top-ups thereafter.' He – and Grace – looked a little disappointed when I said I wasn't sure I have the time. Maybe if ever I decided to retire – the jury definitely out on that one – I might revisit it.

17

DEALING WITH GUILT

'We don't do God' was my throwaway remark to a persistent journalist asking Tony Blair a whole succession of 'just one more question', and this particular 'one final, final question' was 'Prime Minister, tell me about your faith'. 'We don't do God' just popped out of my mouth, became one of those sound bites that stuck, and to this day I get emails and letters from theology and politics students who tell me they are writing their thesis on 'the meaning and strategic thinking behind what you said'. The Archbishop of Canterbury, Justin Welby, I think like my sister, believes one day I will see the light, because he has also asked me to Bible-reading discussions. Of course Tony does do God, famously, but I remain what I call a 'pro-faith atheist', not a believer myself, but respectful and in some ways admiring and slightly jealous of those who do.

But if you don't do God, how do you deal with guilt? I was determined to find a different, more scientific way to deal with the debilitating emotion that is such a major part of depression. I was surprised to discover that the answer might well be found inside an MRI scanner.

I had no idea an MRI scanner was so loud. Despite earplugs better than anything ever given out by cabin crew on an overnight flight, I had to struggle to concentrate in the face of the noise, and for the next stage of my scientific journey, concentration was of the essence.

I was back at the Maudsley in South London, one of the best-known psychiatric hospitals in the world. This time my host was Dr Roland Zahn, reader in mood disorders at the Institute of Psychiatry at King's College London, and we were here to talk about guilt. Mine. He felt it might be a big factor in my depression. Before the anti-Iraq war activists get too excited, this was personal guilt from personal life we were talking about, not political guilt – and of course my depressions pre-dated 9/11, the Taliban in Afghanistan, or the military campaign to bring down Saddam Hussein. I was about to become the forty-fifth guinea pig in a research programme being run by Dr Zahn.

Freud observed when studying grief that some of his patients would go through a healthy grieving process – shock, sadness, fond memories amid the shock and sadness, then recovery of sorts, and life goes on, the pain fades, the fond memories endure. Others, he noticed, would develop depression after losing someone. 'Freud thought the difference was that they blamed themselves, and they felt guilty. It was based on his observations, rather than on a theoretical idea,' Dr Zahn explained.

This struck a chord with me. It is something Liz and I had talked about after Donald died. I am sure he would have said – indeed he did, often – that we were very caring and supportive, and always rushed to help him in a crisis. Yet I felt guilt that there was more I could have done to help him.

When I discussed this with David Sturgeon, he related it to the well-known phenomenon of combat survivor guilt, when soldiers who survive battle are haunted with guilt over those who died. It is one of the factors that lead to suicide among veterans. This was brought home to me recently in Australia where I met the former partner of Jesse Bird, who ended his life on 27 June 2016. 'He joined the Army as a rifleman in 2007,' Connie Boglis told me, 'deployed to Afghanistan in June 2009, returned a different person in February 2010. Ended his life six years later.'

Earlier I had met Darryl Wade, a clinical psychologist who works with veterans. 'Forty-seven Australians lost their lives in combat in Iraq and Afghanistan; 350 have ended their own lives through suicide since coming home. Think how many others are struggling if that is the suicide rate.' Connie, and Jesse Bird's wider family, now campaign non-stop, not just for better services but also to have victims of suicide recognised at the National War Memorial at Canberra.

Unlike Donald, I never served in the military. Yet the 'why him, not me?' question has played on my mind ever since he was diagnosed. It partly explains the terror I felt when psychotic that I was getting the same illness. So was that feeling, that he had been unfairly treated and I had somehow got away with something – survived – a reason for my getting depression in the first place? Was that then exacerbated when it turned out that my fears of schizophrenia, understandable though they were mid-psychotic meltdown, were unfounded? And was the comparison in the lives we went on to lead – mine powerful, high profile, with a strong family of my own; his highly medicated, choices and opportunities limited by his illness, relatively poorly paid, unable to maintain his marriage, childless – a further factor in guilt-driven depression?

Liz, like Tony, like Donald, unlike me, has a deep Christian faith. It is faith not arrogance that leads our sister to say: 'I don't feel guilt at all, and nor should you. We loved him all his life, to the very end. He loved us. He had a good life considering, and he is now in a better place.'

So maybe God helps in more ways than the obvious. But, as you know, I don't do Him, and so that's that. I am not saying that it preys on me the whole time. But I do sometimes have those moments when I ask 'why him, not me?' and when I recall the times I didn't want to have yet another phone call; I didn't want him to come for a weekend I knew was going to be mega-busy; and I didn't care that he thought if only I practised three hours a day, I could get back to competitive standard on the pipes again in a couple of months.

In preparation for the experiment with Dr Zahn, I have to think of two people or things that make me feel guilty. I go for Donald and the kids.

Work and travel often took me away from the children at key moments of their upbringing; and when physically present it wasn't enough. 'What is the point you being here when you're not really here?' Fiona would say. But the children must have been thinking it too. When Rory and Calum were small, and I was pleased they were developing my obsession with football, I would spend Saturdays driving them all the way to Burnley, watching the match, and driving them back again. So, surely, that was being a good dad?

Well, up to a point. As Calum pointed out at one of our family sessions when he was in rehab in Scotland, I spent most of the journey there and back on the phone to politicians and journalists, often bad-tempered, often shouting. There in body, not always in mind. 'Here but not here', Fiona used to call it.

And now I was inside the scanner where Dr Zahn was about to assess how the different parts of my brain communicate to each other, and give me ideas on how to change the way I think. He was focused on how I reacted when 'Donald' and 'kids' flashed up via the mirror I could see at the end of the scanner.

On screens in the control room next door, Dr Zahn watched scans of the parts of my brain relevant to the exercise, the image changing every two seconds. The two regions of the brain he was interested in were the anterior temporal region below the right temple and the depths of the front part of my brain (the subgenual region). 'What I am looking at is how they talk to each other, which we call connectedness.'

The region of the brain below my temple gives the social meaning of my behaviour, whereas the region in the depth of the front part of the brain will tell him if something is 'your fault or not. So if I spill coffee on my shirt, then we think the region below the temple of your brain gives you a detailed interpretation saying this is a sign that I am clumsy, but it actually helps to prevent me from feeling that I'm worthless. And the region here in the depth of the brain would tell me, OK, it is my fault, but being at fault for clumsiness is something I can live with; it's not something that will drive me into a depression. It's all about balance. If one area is over-active or if the two areas are not talking to each other properly, it can make you feel guilty about absolutely everything because it's not receiving the information from the other area of your brain to give you social context. If these brain regions do not talk to each other properly, then you will feel this paralysing form of self-blame; you're blaming yourself for everything without paying attention to the exact nature of the type of behaviour or situation.'

It is similar to when two people talk over each other and the jumble makes no sense. If those two brain parts talk over each other, rather than talk to each other, no independent information gets through.

When I feel guilt about Donald, he says, I probably have no real sense of why I am actually blaming myself. So he challenged me to consider what exactly I'm blaming myself for.

I have instructions to lie very, very still. A number comes up, and my task is to subtract seven from that number, then another seven, then another seven, then another, and so on until the number is replaced by 'kids', or 'Donald', on the screen. The simple mental arithmetic exercise is designed purely as a distraction, forcing me to use different parts of the brain to those I will use when confronted by words likely to make me feel guilty.

When a trigger word comes up, a thermometer gauge measures my emotions. The guiltier I feel, the lower the gauge should be, so my goal is to change the way I am thinking, and drive the gauge upwards.

Strategies used by others in this research programme included accepting things were beyond your control; assessing that the impact was not as bad as feared; apologising; and forgiving yourself or others. This is not just positive thinking. 'That is not really helpful because it would just be repressing self-blame. We want you to genuinely think differently about the guilt, feel a more adaptive, healthier form of guilt. We don't want to wipe away guilt; we just want to get from a depressed guilt to a healthy form of guilt.'

As 'kids' comes up, at first I think of the time in 1994 when Tony had asked me to work for him, and he interrupted our holiday in France to persuade me. Finally, after a month of prevarication, I had said 'yes', and decided to leave Fiona and the children – Grace was just a baby – and head home. Fiona must have mentioned it several hundred times since and, looking back, I can see why. I had made up my mind to take the job and I wanted to get cracking. I announced I would take the car and drive home, so they would need a hire car for the rest of the holiday. So I drove them to the hire car place, said goodbye, headed back to London. Yes, it was just as bad as it sounds. I was in driven mode, nothing could get in the way of what I had decided even though the main reason Fiona had opposed my taking the job in the first place was that it would change her and the children's lives too. So do I feel guilt about that today? I do, especially when I reflect that on my 100 mph-plus charge up the autoroutes I was thinking more about drafting Tony's first Conference speech as leader, talking into a tape recorder as I drove, than whether Fiona was OK with what I was doing. Bad. She had a point.

My challenge is to drive up the gauge and this is the traffic now going through my mind as I lie in the MRI scanner. 'OK, that was bad, no wonder she was pissed off. But come on, you did have to take the job, and Fiona is as Labour as you are, so she ought to be glad we ended up getting rid of the Tories; and OK, we have had ups and downs, but fuck me, we have had a more interesting life than most people. Also, I may not always have been there, but I don't think the kids are in any doubt how much I love them, how I gave whatever spare time I ever had to them, and I know Calum has had the booze issue, Grace has had her issues, but I remember when Rory joined us for that session when Calum was in Castle Craig, the second rehab place he went to, near Peebles, and he said "come on Cam, we had a great childhood, and mum and dad have always been there for us". And you know, maybe they would have had the issues they had whatever we did, who knows, but surely the best thing is to be aware you were never perfect, just keep trying to be better, and make sure they always know you really love them.' The gauge started low, got higher, stayed high for a while, and dipped a bit.

With Donald I found my thoughts were directed not, as above, to myself, but to him. 'Fucking hell, Donald, I wish you were still around. I wish I'd done more for you when you were, but you know, I was often too busy, but you were a great brother, and I hope you think I was too.'

And then, I find myself actually talking back, saying the words out loud, not as me, but as him.

'What the fuck are you on about, Ali? What's all this beating yourself up about me? Listen, I got given a bad deal, OK, but I had a better life than most people with that shitty illness, and one of the reasons was the way the family helped me. Mum and Dad when they were here, you and Liz right to the end, your kids were great to me too, so just shut the fuck up. You were brilliant, son.' The gauge is right at the top, and I hold it there.

A few 'take away seven' exercises later, 'Donald' comes up again, and this time, we're talking about music, and I'm tapping out the notes of a bagpipe tune with my fingers on a rail inside the scanner – disturbing Dr Zahn's data tracking but nonetheless keeping the gauge high. I tell Donald that his best, silver-mounted, ivory pipes are going well, that the ones we gave to the school in Tiree are being well used, and – 'wait for it, I have written a new tune'.

'Go on, play it.'

So I do, and he hums along, and the gauge stays high. It is a tactic I have used since, without the need to clamber inside a scanner.

Of course guilt and self-blame are important for the functioning of society. 'We need guilt in order to promote our behaving well. Psychopaths are guilt-free. A society free of guilt is a society full of psychopaths.' On the other hand, Dr Zahn says, 'people with depression tend to overgeneralise guilt, so they feel guilty for everything, rather than a specific thing. What we're trying to do with the study is promote a healthy mean of a sense of guilt that doesn't paralyse you but allows you to act on your feelings of guilt.'

When I am in depressive ruminating mode, I can very quickly switch from guilt about my absence when the kids were small to what was the point of it all anyway because I didn't stay the course, we lost the election after I left though I went back to help – too little, too late. If I had gone back earlier, could I have stopped David Cameron from winning, and if I had, no Brexit, if no Brexit maybe no Trump, if no Trump we could deal with climate change, but Trump is there, climate change is real, so it is my fucking fault the world is going to end. And if I am in anger/guilt mode rather than pure guilt mode, I might say to Fiona: 'You do realise the world is ending and it's because you stopped me working in Number 10.'

This is madness in a way, but also compelling evidence of how the brain can spiral into all sorts of weird places. When I am anxious and insomniac, I can waste literally an hour of my life agonising about how many shirts and how many wire hangers to take on an upcoming overseas trip, all woven around with fears about the world ending. Yet my most creative periods will often come immediately after one of those nights.

In the Freudian model, anger is turned inwards, making the depressed mind feel more guilty, blaming itself more, but Dr Zahn adds: 'People also feel angry towards others as a defence mechanism when they blame themselves, and that can turn into a vicious cycle.' He calls it 'the guilt indignation cycle, where you blame yourself for something you've done; you try to make yourself feel better by trying to direct the blame at others, to feel angry towards them, and then you feel bad about yourself again for doing this. So it's very different from antisocial people who just feel predatory anger. What we're trying to do is to break through that cycle by trying to diminish self-blame. And we are also trying to help people to feel angry at others when it's appropriate to do so, because what we've found is that people with depression have a diminished sense of anger. That is a problem because they can't stand up for themselves. Some people have told us after the study that they're now better able to stand up for themselves.

'There is an interesting overlap here with bipolar disorder. People feel more irritable and angry towards others when they get into a high. So there is a theory that people with irritability and depression might be more similar to those with bipolar disorder than unipolar depression, and that's a very interesting research question. To me, major depression is a set of very consistent symptoms, the most important of which is feeling bad about yourself, feeling worthless. That sense of worthlessness can only be explained if you blame yourself for things that have gone wrong in your life. If you don't blame yourself for the things that go wrong in your life, you don't feel bad about yourself; you feel bad about the world but not about yourself. To me, that is the key to understanding depression.'

So blaming myself for Donald's schizophrenia, or Calum's alcoholism, or the world ending, or Burnley losing a game because I missed it, is only likely to apply if and when I am feeling worthless, and blaming myself for things not totally under my control. He distinguishes between 'healthy blame' – you do something you know is wrong, you make amends, you learn – and 'unhealthy blame' where you take responsibility also for things you didn't do or couldn't control. 'Blaming yourself for Donald is a good example of unhealthy guilt, because you cannot be responsible for him having a severe mental illness. It is the kind of thing people with depression often feel, and it is survivor guilt.'

Dr Zahn points out that in his native language, German, which was also Freud's, guilt and blame are the same word – *Schuld*. 'It's only in English that there is this difference,' he says. 'But there's also a theoretical view that self-blame is cognitive and guilt is emotional, whereas to me that doesn't really make sense. I think that the cognitive elements and the emotional elements are so linked together that you can't separate them.'

Later, I rerun the footage of Dr Zahn watching the images of my brain as they are fed to him every two seconds. He reminds me of a football commentator, intense, quiet at times, monotone at others, then suddenly excited as he sees something he thinks is happening that will help his research.

Dr ZAHN: This graph is a measure of the crosstalk between the two brain regions, and as the patient uses the strategies, look, the crosstalk goes down, and this is a success, and that's what we feed back to him with the thermometer scale. It has nothing to do with temperature: it reflects the level of crosstalk in his brain as we measure it. So the thermometer level goes up if we want to signal success to Alastair. This is new stuff – we're seeing neuro-feedback information from people's own brains coming back to them in real time.

So this is a specific scan which shows the connections between the two brain regions that we're interested in. So here, you can see the connection, the cable bundle that connects the temple region with the front part. And the cables conveying the electrical signals are carried through this bundle. These cable connections are absolutely key in helping us to train people to feel differently about guilt, people with depression. Many people think about the brain as something you can't change, but that's not true because our brain changes all the time; every time we learn something, the connections in our brains change.

Now . . . ah, the thermometer is going down, so obviously the strategy has not worked. Now, he's been able to bring it full up, so he seems to have a strategy that works again. But you can see that he's moved more, so probably because it was emotionally quite involved, he started to move without noticing. Now, here we go, Donald, guilt-related scenario. He's getting feedback based on the baseline and he's at the bottom . . . OK, he's now starting to play around with the strategies. But it seems to be quite hard right now for him to get out of this high correlation. But he's actually . . . Yeah, in the strategy he's currently following, it doesn't work. He's moved even further, the crosstalk even higher . . . Ah, now, it's worked, so he's bringing the level of correlation down. Now look, he's done something that really works, so he should get this idea now, OK, something I'm doing right now is working, continues to work every two seconds, and he can see that on the thermometer. So now he's held it, good . . . OK, now he's got to work on the subtraction again. But I hope that he will remember what he's done in the last block and then once he's finished with the subtraction, he can continue to do this. OK, here we go, Donald again. So he can work with the same scenario. It should make it easier for him to employ the same strategies. The thing is, he will have a new baseline, won't he? So we could actually make it more difficult because we're starting from a different correlation level. So let's see how he's doing. So he seems to do well in keeping the correlation level at the lower end of the range. So he's done that . . . Wow, look, yeah, he found the strategy, and that was instantaneous, wasn't it? Wow. See!

Now he's going back to subtracting sevens. His baseline correlation for 'kids' is actually lower than 'Donald', which means he's already employing the strategies to that scenario while we're acquiring the baseline measure. OK, now he's found it again. So he's done something, it's either the same strategy or another strategy. But his correlation levels are creeping up, that's why he gets a feedback that he's not doing the right thing. So it's interesting. He really needs to work hard. It seems that if he doesn't work hard, the correlation goes up, the thermometer comes down.

Then a little later: 'I think he's doing very consistently. He seems to have found something that works – a strategy that works for him for both scenarios, "kids" and "Donald". That's important, because we want people to use those strategies for everyday life.'

Out of the experiment, they have made a 3D print of my brain, which is to be exhibited as part of a Wellcome Trust project on neuroscience and art. I am surprised to discover that a phrase I am fond of using about clever people – 'they have a brain the size of a planet' – is meaningless. When it comes to brains, he tells me, size doesn't matter. It is all about how the cells operate. As for how I felt at the end of it, the honest answer is exhausted, and shocked to discover that though my pulse is usually in the high 40s/low 50s, at one point, presumably when really fighting to push that thermometer higher, it shot up to over 100. I said afterwards that I was once told I suffered from 'maladaptive competitiveness', and explained, laughing: 'Whenever the thermometer came down . . . I felt very disappointed in myself.'

MRI scanners are neither cheap nor plentiful, but Dr Zahn is hopeful the thinking behind this neuro-feedback research programme will eventually lead to a version of it being available on our phones, or via infra-red, easily accessible, easily used. He feels this kind of treatment might work better than CBT – which I have tried twice, without the success others have reported.

'The thing with CBT is that it still relies on a relationship between the therapist and a client working through what they call the Socratic dialogue with yourself. It's basically the therapist asks questions so that you question some of your assumptions, and by the end of the therapy you're supposed to ask these questions yourself and have that Socratic dialogue with yourself. The problem is often that people don't even remember what they've done in CBT because it's very complex. This is relatively simple. So people will be able to remember one or two strategies that have worked for them. That is easier to implement on a day-to-day basis.' I buy that. And I have definitely benefited from the tactic of talking to myself and to others in my imagination whenever feelings of survivor guilt, or any other form of guilt, kick in.

18

IN THE BLOOD

I was a little worried about the next leg of my scientific journey. First, because it involved needles and blood, both of which I am abnormally sensitive to and have caused me to faint all too often in the past. Three incidents in particular spring to mind: the time I recalled earlier, when I collapsed at the sight of a body in Devon and Cornwall Police HQ; the time Fiona, when pregnant with Grace, had to have an amniocentesis test and I went along to support her, not realising it involved the insertion of a giant needle into her pregnancy bump – cue fainting, and the nurses looking after her suddenly having to look after me on the floor; and then the time Rory was in A&E having fallen and smashed his head, I rushed to his bedside after being called by the hospital, promptly fainted on seeing needles and drips being put into him, and was immediately put into the neighbouring bed and kept in overnight for observation.

The Maudsley had taken a sample of my blood and sent it to Dr Golam Khandaker, a Fellow of Cambridge University's Institute of Psychiatry. I am today certainly in better physical shape than when I was there as a student, yet I never like being given the results of real medical tests, which in this case were seeking to establish levels of inflammation, which are linked to depression.

Dr Khandaker admitted, based on what he knew about me, that he was expecting to give me news I might not want to hear – not of imminent death, but that years of dissolute living followed by decades of high-stress work might have left me with what could be termed bad blood. He knew I had been a heavy drinker and smoker, and that I had only committed to regular exercise once I was into my forties. He knew that I had had a chronic inflammatory physical illness, ulcerative colitis, diagnosed in the mid-1990s during a period of high (pre-election) stress, for which I took medication for many years and which I was told was likely to stay with me indefinitely, and possibly morph into Crohn's Disease. He said that a stressful job and the pressures of a public profile were also risk factors likely to have caused higher levels of inflammation.

But my blood is good. My protein levels are just right. Based on this analysis, he tells me, I am in 'the most healthy group of people in the country'. If I had continued with my heavy drinking, smoking, bad diet, no exercise, taking little concern over sleep, the chances are the inflammation would have been worse, much worse, possibly dangerously so. In addition to the other physical health effects, that would have impacted on my depression for the worse too. This made me think of my brother Graeme.

'The positive thing here', he says, 'is that you have taken decisions about the way you live which have benefited your physical and your mental health. You have controlled the risk factors and brought the inflammation levels down.' It might also explain why my ulcerative colitis had miraculously vanished a few years ago when I went for an all too regular colonoscopy.

'Our brain sits within the body,' he explains, 'so the separation between mind and body is unhelpful.' So I am signed up totally to the view that mental and physical health are two sides of the same coin. Like most non-medics, I suspect, if someone says inflammation, I think of fever, or a swelling, a harsh redness perhaps. That, he says, is acute, high-level inflammation, a normal response in our body, essential for survival, to fight off infection. But in some people, the immune system operates as though fighting off an infection all the time. 'It is like a thermostat always cranked up to a slightly higher temperature,' he says, 'and this low-grade inflammation is harmful for a number of physical and psychiatric illnesses, such as depression and heart disease.'

His team did a study of 5,000 children from the Greater Bristol area, measuring their level of inflammation when they were nine years old, and psychiatric symptoms when they were eighteen. A higher level of inflammation in childhood was associated with increased risk of developing depression and psychosis when they were young adults. He cites that as possible evidence that inflammation may not be simply a consequence of illness, but a cause.

He points to flu, or even the common cold, as an illustration of the link between our immune system and our mood. 'When we have flu we feel depressed, not very sociable, can't think properly, and these are also common symptoms of depression. Also, some patients with depression show increased levels of inflammation, but again we don't know for sure whether that's a consequence of illness or a cause.'

In addition to bad lifestyle choices and psychological stress, early life adversity and trauma can set the immune system on a path of chronic activity. So dealing with the trauma, and addressing smoking, excessive alcohol, unhealthy diet and obesity, all of which are linked with inflammation, do help increase mental wellbeing.

Alcohol has a potent, often positive effect on our mood, short term. It can make us feel more confident and happier. So someone with depression might drink to feel better, to drown their sorrows; someone with anxiety, for Dutch courage. But the long-term effects send the mood in a very different direction: downwards. As he talks, I am thinking again of my chats with Dr Bennie in Ross Hall Hospital in Paisley. Throwing up, hangovers, the shakes . . . I don't need persuading that excessive drinking contributes to both physical and psychiatric problems.

A third of patients with depression do not respond very well to antidepressants, and a third of patients with depression show evidence of inflammation. He believes that is no coincidence, because inflammation is one of the causes of some patients failing to respond to antidepressants. But what Dr Khandaker's current work shows is that patients with chronic inflammatory physical illness who take anti-inflammatory drugs have also seen improvement in any depression or depressive symptoms they might have been displaying. Unlike Dr Moncrieff, he does see a continuing role for antidepressants in treating a large group of patients with depression. But, especially for those who fail to respond to antidepressants or psychological therapies, anti-inflammatories could well be a part of a treatment. 'I don't think the anti-inflammatory is the ultimate solution for all people with depression,' he says. 'But it could well provide another tool for treating people with depression.'

19

IS DEPRESSION GENETIC?

The next stop on my journey was Toronto to meet the founder of the world's first specialist psychiatric genetic counselling clinic, Dr Jehannine Austin. I was hoping she could help with the 'why me?' questions. Why do I get depression? Why did Donald get schizophrenia? Was there anything in our family background that could have alerted us to Lachie's suicide, and helped us to prevent it? Whether, in short, our illnesses are embedded in our genes.

Dr Austin had travelled from British Columbia to meet me, and I was immediately struck by her warmth. She also immediately came over as practical and full of common sense. She asked very direct questions and in minutes I found myself sharing my life story and my innermost feelings, and it all felt totally natural.

She likes visuals. She likes images, and soon she was taking what I was saying and turning it into what she calls my 'genetic map'. Men are squares, women are circles, and so we started with a large square – me – right at the heart of the page. My parents were added above, my siblings alongside me, then aunts and uncles, cousins, nieces and nephews. She was interested in anything related to psychological and psychiatric issues, theirs and mine, as well as the impact of theirs on mine.

Where there was a mild medical issue, she shaded lightly in the corner of the square or circle of the person affected; where it was serious, as with Donald and Lachie, she filled it in more deeply. In my map, for example, depression got heavy shading and anxiety a few dots, and she scribbled notes alongside. Where I was unsure about more distant family, she put a question mark.

Once we had done my family background, we went into Fiona's family tree to work out the genetic map for our children, part of the exercise being to check out their vulnerability as well as my own. There is a bit of alcoholism, a bit of depression, but in the main her side is healthier than mine. 'If Fiona had experienced mental health problems as well,' Dr Austin explained, 'the chances for your children would be elevated. As a general rule, the greater the number of people in the family who have experienced problems, and the more closely related they are to the people for whom we're calculating chances, the higher the chances are going to be.'

So, take Lachie, for example. As my cousin, he is four steps of the bloodline away from my children – step 1 me, step 2 my Dad, step 3 his brother, uncle Hector, step 4 Lachie – and she would argue therefore that the genetic impact on them is minimal.

I told her that just as I worried when I had psychosis that I was developing schizophrenia, so Grace feared the same when she was having panic attacks in Paris. She had always been fascinated by 'Donald's voices' and developed an unhealthy fear she was heading the same way.

Dr Austin's assessment of my map suggested 'a little bit of increased genetic vulnerability to mental illness for our children'. But also, she was keen to stress, even if somebody inherits a lot of genetic vulnerability, that doesn't mean that they're destined to get sick. It just allows us to be aware of the risks and that can be helpful. I should also be aware, she tells me, that if a parent has had a significant mental health problem – as I did aged twenty-nine – that age can become an important milestone for the child, who might feel more vulnerable around that time. Again, useful information, even if you do nothing with it.

The relative lack of squiggles next to the square and the circle representing my parents, alongside the mass of information she is putting alongside Donald, Graeme, Liz and me, is startling. I am reminded of something my nephew Graeme Naish, Liz's son, said to my parents once: 'How come you two, normal as they come, produced these four nutters?'

It was a fair question. My Dad might have had periods in his life when he drank too much, but he was not an alcoholic. He might have been grouchy at times, but I don't believe he was a depressive. As for my Mum, I don't think I have ever known a happier person. As

Rory said when she died, he had no memory of her in a bad mood, remembered her always smiling, laughing, singing or humming. Donald's illness, as I said earlier, was a big turning point in her life, but it did not change her basic outlook – that life was good, people were lovely, there was no detail in anyone's life that was not worth talking about, and it was always important to look on the bright side and see the good in people, places and things. It must have been hard for someone so clearly not affected by mental illness to have so much of it to deal with in her immediate family.

I told Dr Austin a recurring conversation my mother and I had many times down the years.

'Ali,' she would say, 'why can't you just be content?'

'What does content mean?'

'Satisfied with what you have.'

'Ah, complacent?'

'No. Not complacent. Content.'

'You mean boring then?'

'No. Content.'

'Sounds like complacent and boring to me.'

When she died, and we were sitting around chatting about her, friends and relatives wandering into my sister's house, someone asked everyone to say one word that they felt summed up my Mum.

'Happy' came top by a mile. Yet there too I think our views were very different. I see contentment as compla-cency and happiness not as a state of mind, but a goal, something that we should pursue in our life over time, and indeed that we will only really know if we have lived a happy life as we near its end. As I explained earlier, this may be the atheist's way of staying broadly on the straight and narrow, I don't know. But whenever I expressed this view to my Mum she would shake her head, suggest I was 'bonkers, Ali', and go and make yet another cup of tea.

Fiona once declared content to be 'Alastair's least favourite word in the English language', and though I loved my Mum dearly, and miss her smiling face and sing-song voice, it is true. She saw her role as a mother and a housewife, a nurturer and protector, and, especially after Donald was diagnosed and had to leave the Army, I think those protective instincts grew.

Though she was very proud of what I did in politics, she really wished I wasn't doing it. This was so much the case that she stopped reading newspapers, and yet had stacks of cuttings about me in her bottom drawer, brought to her by neighbours, most chucked unread, the nicer ones cut out and pasted lovingly into a collection of scrapbooks we only found after she died.

Whenever I was particularly under the cosh, she would avoid TV and radio. Despite having barely any fat on her, she would lose lots of weight when I was really under pressure and getting lambasted across politics and the media. When Tony once phoned when I was visiting her, I put him on for a chat, told him to tell her to stop worrying about me. They talked away nicely about this, that and the other, him charming, her nice and supportive, but then she said: 'Anyway, Tony, lovely to talk to you, but I'll hand you back to Ali now.

I need to go to the loo . . . his working for you tends to give me diarrhoea!'

It was partly the impact of my profile that made her want me not to talk about Donald in public, even though he was the reason I campaigned on mental health. Donald was keen to be out there too, which is why we had talked about making a film about his schizophrenia. But the thought of it filled her with panic and dread.

When finally I left Number 10, I think she hoped I would somehow retire. 'Ali, why on earth are you going to New Zealand? Can you not just be content at home?'

As we talk, Dr Austin starts to notice patterns. There are certainly more squiggles on my Dad's side of the family, what with drink, and gambling problems among sons, brothers, uncles and cousins, depressions and anxieties too. While my Mum's family was largely teetotal, and largely, it must be said, 'content', there is one big mental health story that has been weighing down on me. It concerns my maternal grandfather's sister.

Of her five children, two killed themselves, while two of the remaining three had ECT for depression. That is heavy. But Dr Austin isn't even adding this to the map. 'I'm not going to draw them in because from a genetic standpoint, they're too distantly related to you. Once you get past a third-degree relative, the genetic variations you share are less and less, so the chance of it increasing your own probability of developing illness just disappears.'

She explains that basically for every single line drawn we lose about fifty per cent of the shared genetic information between individuals in the family. 'So from the perspective of how you are impacted by that, if I was to draw them out, they would be off the map.' God, I wish I had met her ages ago. That family story had long hung over me.

That morning, knowing I would be raising this double family suicide with Dr Austin, I called another of Mum's cousins, Sheena Downie, to make sure I had the facts right. Sheena, who has also had issues with depression and anxiety – 'Sheena's nerves are not so good today,' my Mum used to put it – said something very telling about the suicides and the ECT in her family. 'The thing was, at the time, you just didn't talk about it.' How much harder that must have made things. It leaves me with an overwhelming feeling of sadness, and waste for everyone involved, but also strengthens my determination to fight stigma and taboo. The more we normalise mental illness, the better we can deal with it.

Dr Austin notices another pattern, in how I was expressing myself when talking about all these issues we are mapping, whether it is my own depression, Donald's schizophrenia, Graeme's unaddressed depression or addictions, Calum's or my uncle James's alcoholism, my niece Kate's hemiplegia – or Lachie's suicide.

'Every time you talk about these things, I have a sense of your feeling of helplessness. You want to fix it all. You want to take control or have power over it, and when you can't, you feel helpless in the face of it, and that feels like a big challenge.' She has got to the nub of my depression in half an hour.

I am a self-confessed control freak, and in my professional and political life I have often been able to exercise that control, by working hard, by being committed and dedicated, and developing systems, teams and contacts to help me regulate the space in which I operate. And perhaps this is easier in work, especially if you have a propensity for long hours and packing a lot into them, than it is in our emotional life and, even more so, the emotional life of others.

I do have a tendency to think I can fix not just my own problems but other people's too. And often I can. But it means that when I discover that actually I can't – I couldn't stop Donald being ill, I couldn't persuade Calum not to drink, I couldn't stop Grace panicking on the Paris Metro, I wasn't even aware that Lachie might be about to kill himself as he phoned Donald that day, I later learned, not me – yet I somehow feel responsible.

These things are all in my space, they are right there on my genetic map, and there is nothing I can do about any of them. I want to fix it all, but despite being the guy who is supposed to be able to fix things, I can't. That feels like a personal failure and I take it as such. This can quickly lead to feelings of helplessness morphing into worthlessness, and my depressive spiral kicks in once more.

What Dr Austin says about my need for control chimes with something said by the person who knows me better than anyone else alive. Fiona cited a journalist who used to travel with Tony and me once telling her: 'I've never seen anyone like Alastair in terms of the way he could walk into a room and command the space around him.' She thinks I have got that power and that I like to have it, to know I can control the people around me despite the fact that it can be quite difficult to live with.

Dr Austin suggests you should think of your life as a jam jar. For this visual, she uses yellow balls – as genetic factors – and yellow triangles – as environmental or experiential factors. She drops the yellow balls into the jar. These are our genes. They are the sediment in the jar. There is nothing we can do about them. They are accidents of birth dependent on our parents and other relatives.

Depression is not like, for example, Huntington's disease where if the parent has that particular gene it is passed on to the child. The mind is different. If there is mental illness in that sediment, from the experiences of our relatives, it is not guaranteed we will inherit it. There is no single gene variation that we've yet found that is either necessary or sufficient in order for somebody to develop a psychiatric illness. 'It is not that genetics is not important to psychiatric illness. Genetics is very important to psychiatric illness, but it's not the only thing. There is no single gene that predicts you will have schizophrenia, depression or OCD.'

There are a huge number of different genetic variations that can increase a person's vulnerability to developing one of these disorders. 'We all have some genetic vulnerability to mental illness.' We need to live with the sediment. It is what it is. Any genetic vulnerability is there for life and there is nothing we can do to change it. Those yellow balls sit, unmoving, at the bottom of the jam jar. 'I think the most important thing to know in general is that mental illness is not your fault, it's not anyone's fault. It just is.'

The rest of the jar is our life, filled with good experiences and bad. Good memories and bad. Into the jar, then out, go things we learn, but forget. More likely to stay are things we learn and remember. This can start as early as the pregnancy of your mother. There may be a causal link between a difficult birth and developing mental illness in early adulthood. 'We know that people who develop schizophrenia in later life have a higher probability of having been delivered in circumstances that were complicated. They may have been more likely to have the cord wrapped around their neck.' Likewise, she goes on, 'childhood head injuries can add vulnerability to the jar', and I think immediately of the time – I was too young to remember but it became one of those family stories – when I was dropped in the bath. Then there's the time my Auntie Grace swung a golf club not realising Graeme was behind her and took a chunk out of his forehead; and the time Calum came off his bike, crashing head first into a railing on Hampstead Heath.

If the mind gets too full and unable to process everything in there in a healthy, sustaining way, there is a risk it will explode into illness. But our family genetic map, with a lot less happening on Fiona's side than mine, suggests our children have less genetic vulnerability than I did.

As human beings, as parents, you want the very best for your kids all of the time. But we can't select the genes that we pass on. While these variations may increase their vulnerability to mental illness, they can be associated just as much with traits we value, such as empathy, creativity, compassion and resilience. It is important not to frame it all as negative.

Dr Austin was again reassuring. 'When we look at the genetic background, the effects are general not specific. If there is depression and schizophrenia in the background, it doesn't mean you are likelier to get those; it might mean a general susceptibility but it could emerge as OCD or anxiety.'

'When the jam jar is full?'

'Exactly.'

'So there are no empty jars in the world?'

'None.'

'The Pope does not have an empty jar.'

'There are no empty jars.'

'The Archbishop of Canterbury does not have an empty jar.'

'Correct.'

'In fact I know he doesn't. He told me about his issues with depression, and his daughter's.'

'No empty jam jars. None. All a matter of degree.'

*

Life needs to take its course. Where we cannot change the yellow circles, we can change the triangles. So Calum no longer drinks, and that means a very large triangle has gone. Grace used to smoke a lot of weed – both cannabis and crystal meth have been shown to increase vulnerability to mental illness – but now doesn't, so her jam jar is emptier than it was, though it will have other pressures – it's not easy making it as a stand-up comedian – to crowd into the vacated space. The fact that our three children have seen so much mental illness in others close to them could actually be a help in that they will feel more able to be open, and have a better idea if and when help might be needed, and know how to get it.

We spend an awful lot of time analysing our genes and sitting down with therapists to go over our past. But this is looking at things in the wrong way. 'You cannot undo the jam jar,' she says. 'But you can grow it. You can add layers, protective factors, rings stacking on top of the jar, making it taller so it can accommodate more environmental or experiential stuff and give you more space in which to manage your life.'

Stress can be both good and bad, depending on how we handle it. Being creative, being empathetic – qualities that may come from mania or depression – can help create more space in the jar. The joy of this approach, she says, is that whereas with physical illness we all tend to get pretty much the same treatments, with this we can make our own.

20

THE LIFE-SAVING JAM JAR

A few nights later, back home in London, my conscious and my subconscious clearly chatting in my sleep, I awake with a light bulb going off in my head. It is 3.35 a.m. Fiona is asleep. I get up, walk down to the kitchen, sit with pen and paper, and draw my jam jar.

There is the jar, short and squat. There is the sediment, the yellow balls, filling maybe a fifth of it, packed into the bottom of the jar. And here is my life, good and bad, remembered and forgotten, chaotic scribbles, it is all mixed up, but one thing is for sure: I have packed a lot in, so no wonder there have been explosions from time to time. So what Dr Austin was telling me is that I can talk all I want about what is *in* the jar. But I cannot undo it. What I just need to do is *grow* the jam jar instead.

I start with the large additional layer, which turns out to be the biggest of them all. I call it FFF – Fiona, family and friends. These are the relationships that truly matter. In that order. If Fiona and I are strong, our family is strong. If we are getting on, my life is so much better than when we do not. My decision-making is better. My productivity is higher. My moods are much, much better if she and I are good together. And if my moods are better, I am likely to be a better parent, less wrapped up in my own mind, struggles, ambitions or pleasure. If the children are happy, I am happy. I cannot dictate their happiness but I can contribute to it, or detract from it. So I must work hard to contribute, knowing that I won't always succeed. I must make sure they know I love them more than any other people on earth. Stay in close touch with my wider family, too, especially Liz. If you value your real friends, you know the difference between true friends and the hundreds of others in your orbit. Be there for them, and they will be there for you.

Next up, the second biggest slab added to my jam jar, is meaningful activity. I draw a dotted line going through it, to signal two parts, paid and unpaid. I like to have cash in my pocket. It is why I loved busking as a young man. I like to feel that if I suddenly want to travel somewhere, or buy something, I can.

I want to be comfortable. But I also need meaningful activity. According to Fiona, especially when I am a bit manic, my first words of the day, literally on waking up, can often be 'so how am I going to change the world today?' And sometimes my meaningful activity is paid. This book won't make me rich but it might help change the way some look at mental health. It might change the mind of a government minister, or a future government minister. It might inspire someone to go into psychiatry or to seek help. I hope so.

Then we are into what I call the general practicals. Diet. Eat well, avoid crap, watch the booze. Sleep well. Exercise often. Everyone should think of those, and their relation to our wellbeing.

Next is the personal. For me a big part of that is BFC. Burnley Football Club is a hugely important part of my wellbeing. Football connects me to a bigger community, close to my roots. It gives me highs and lows, and wonderful memories of triumph and setback alike.

Fiona has never really been able to understand the Burnley thing. She tried for a while, but what do you do with someone you take to a game and she asks when 'the interval' is and, once 'the interval' is over, why the teams have swapped shirts? But then I don't understand why she loves opera so much, and is so keen for me to go along, even though I am likely merely to have a very expensive sleep.

Football gives me something I am always looking forward to – the next match, the next season. It has given me a circle of friends and acquaintances separate from my daily life in London: the fans I meet home and away; the staff at the club; the board, several of whom have become friends, two of the managers especially, Stan Ternent and Sean Dyche; players present and past, like Paul Fletcher, who has become a close friend and with whom I have done business, written a novel and performed, me with my bagpipes, him with his ukulele, in old folks' homes. Wheels within wheels again. The circles of life.

The world is not going to be that much better or worse if we win or don't win against Crystal Palace, yet in the moment it matters so much; that sense of – particularly when we score – completely losing yourself in the moment with all these other people. When we played at Leicester last year, I didn't realise that a photographer was taking my picture as I was celebrating a goal, and there were photos in one of the papers where I'm literally jumping all over this guy who's next to me. I haven't got a clue who he is. My sister jokes with me that she has real religion but Burnley is mine, and it's true that singing a football chant with thousands of other people speaks to something in me I don't get anywhere else. What a lot of people get in a church, I get at a football match, and when things go really, really well, it's great, it's a fantastic feeling.

That brings me nicely to music, another big part of the jam jar. I love music so much and I love so much music. Listening to it, playing it, writing it. I love music that makes me happy, makes me sad, makes me cry, makes me think. And sometimes I can feel all four things in one single session on the pipes. Jacques Brel, Elvis or Edith Piaf can do all four better than anyone. I never tire of listening to them.

Then creativity, whether writing, or campaigning, or having ideas and making them happen. Attached to that is curiosity, always staying curious, reading, exploring, seeing whatever we do as work in progress, perfection unattainable, new goals always to be set and reached, new ideas to be enjoyed, now reinforced by Roland Zahn's observation that our brain changes every time we learn something new. And not forgetting the natural world: beautiful scenery can always shift my mood, usually for the better.

And here is the thing – if you had been sitting next to me on the outward flight to Toronto to meet Dr Austin, and you had said to me, 'hope you don't mind me asking, but I read you have depression, and I just wanted to ask how you dealt with it to be able to live the life you do', I might have replied: 'Well, I take pills every day and I see a shrink when things are really shit.' But when I created my jam jar, David and sertraline came last, not first, after all the other protective rings. My jam jar has given me a new way of thinking about myself, about my depression, about life. And it has certainly helped me to live better.

I discovered more about the science underlying this from a clinical psychologist working for the NHS in Edinburgh, Massimo Tarsia. He said the jam jar is a simple illustration of a well-known 'stress-vulnerability' model, with genetic (circles) and environmental (triangles) vulnerabilities filling up the jar. 'The jar extension rings represent all the positive lifestyle changes you have been able to make over the years which help you be more resilient,' he said. He added that there is a limit to the amount of rings we can add to our jam jars. In addition to building protective factors, it is important to attend to those triangles that keep filling up the jar, in case they become too heavy to carry around with us, so that they spill over and become impossible to bear.

He emphasised that these need not be major stressors or traumatic life events, the so-called 'dark secrets of the past', but could simply be the gradual build-up of more minor stressors, which develop into something bigger. There is rarely an obvious trigger for a depressive episode. 'Childhood adversity is a common factor in depression, but this does not necessarily mean extreme forms of abuse. It is more often the case that the cumulative experience of difficult early relationships, and the learning from these, interferes with normal cognitive and emotional development and eventually – with the accumulation of triangles – leads to the development of depression. That is why, in therapy for depression, the aim is to make sense of the likely reasons for the development of depression, and to review and change the way we deal with situations in our daily life.'

He explained a relatively new treatment, CBASP, which stands for Cognitive Behavioural Analysis System of Psychotherapy. He said it was the only psychological therapy specifically developed to treat persistent depression. Next on my list, perhaps, if I slip back into regular periods of struggle. For sure, I am resigned to having them.

Indeed, a few months after drawing my jam jar in the early hours at the kitchen table, after a pretty long run of good health, I had a particularly bad plunge. As so often, it came on holiday, when we had gone with friends and family to the Highlands of Scotland, the highlight of which I described earlier, when we celebrated Fiona's sixtieth birthday. It was a wonderful night, and though I was tired the next day, I had no sense of the impending cloud that was to crowd in on me. This time, unusually, it first made itself known to me not on waking, but as I began to feel some symptoms gathering as the day continued. And then suddenly, as we were all sitting round for dinner, almost like a switch being turned on, I was not OK at all. Some of our best-loved friends were there, people we have known for a long time. I was fine one moment, and then in the next, I was anything but. It was a spectacular, terrifying crash. I tried to keep eating, but now the food had no taste.

One of our oldest friends, someone we have known since *Tavistock Times* days, Carolyn Fairbairn, now the head of the CBI, was talking to me about Brexit, and I was going through the motions, knowing I was failing to engage. As our friends around the room began to notice something was seriously wrong, Fiona felt she had to raise it. She asked me if I was OK, but by then I was plunging so far and so fast I could not speak, so I just shook my head a little, less to say I wasn't OK than 'don't bother me, carry on as though I am not here, don't worry about me'. But given they all know I can get severely depressed, not worrying is a lot easier for me to say than for them to do, and I felt my mood dragging the whole room down. I stood up. I had to leave immediately, and went to find somewhere to hide. I had a desperate desire to be invisible, not to be there, not to have to share the emptiness or make anyone feel they had to know it or understand it or be part of it. It is the most dreadful, desolate feeling that you cannot explain, and if you try, it only serves to make you feel worse, because the effort drags you further down the spiral. One minute I was fine, the next I was hollowed out, not even listening to anything being said, not caring, not eating, not anything; alive in that I was breathing, but feeling totally dead inside. Dead and alive at the same time. That is how it feels. That is how it felt that night, and there was nothing I could do about it.

'Are you aware of the power you have over other people's emotions when that happens?' Fiona asked the next day.

'No,' I said. 'I am aware of my utter power*lessness* to do anything about it, and it makes me feel absolutely wretched.'

'Mmmm, OK.'

But this time – hiding in a farm outhouse in the Scottish Highlands, feeling terrible that I had walked away from Fiona, family and friends, knowing that their lively chatter would have gradually resumed after I left but that the shadow my mood had cast would still be present – I had gone from three or four on my scale in the morning to six or seven, and now nine, and suddenly thinking rather dangerously about ten. I was leaning against a wall, sitting on a stone floor. It was so cold. I thought perhaps if I just walked up the glen at the back of the house, and kept going till I collapsed, perhaps I would just freeze to death. Or I might stumble and fall in the dark, break a limb, and let the cold take me that way, unable to move. These were scary flights of fancy. They passed.

As I came back closer to eight, I sent Fiona a text to say I was fine, I just needed a bit of time on my own, and would see her in bed in a while. 'OK x,' she replied. That was fine. I knew she would go into a bit of a shutdown, because part of how she now handles my plunges is no longer to blame herself but to be there for me if I want her to be, and not if I don't.

I decided I would only go back to the house once I was confident everyone was in bed and Fiona would be asleep – I settled on 2 a.m. – but then, as I started to worry I might not last that long without going to get some extra clothes or blankets, Jehannine's jam jar – or my version of it – popped into my head, and I made a plan. I decided that come the morning, I would take my jam jar and work through it, doing something related to everything I had added to it after my trip to Toronto.

And I did. The first step was to be open with Fiona, Family and Friends. At breakfast the next morning, I did something I had never done before. I waited till everyone was up, and I apologised to them all for my depression, or at least explained that I understood this had had an impact not just on me, but on them too.

'I just wanted to say something about last night,' I said. 'I don't know why, but I had a sudden massive plunge. I had been feeling it coming on, I tried to stave it off, but the tipping point came as we were having dinner, and I was gone. I am sorry if it ruined your evening.' At which point Tessa Jowell, herself at the time fighting the tumour that would kill her, stood up, came over, hugged me tightly and said 'we know, and we love you all the more for it'. And Fiona smiled at me, although she never lets herself get carried away with the idea that this would be the last time this kind of thing happened.

And then, over the course of the following hours, I worked my way through the rest of the jar.

Meaningful Activity. I worked on a speech I was due to give the next week in Germany, which was about crisis management as it happens, and I now decided to add a section on personal as well as corporate and governmental crisis management, and on the importance of resilience.

Exercise. I still felt like shit but Fiona and I went for a long walk and a long talk, and later I went for a short run. It was a struggle, but I felt better for it.

Burnley. I called Sean Dyche for a chat about the game against Huddersfield. He knows about my depression and we often talk about it in relation to sport, sports psychology and performance maximisation. He humours me by pretending to take my analysis of players and teams seriously. But he does take the chats we have about mental health seriously.

'I've had ups and downs like everyone,' he says, 'but not the way you talk about it. But I feel I need to know about it. If you think how many people work for a Premier League football club, by the law of averages there are going to be a fair few with some sort of issue, and we need to know how to handle it, how to help.'

Music. I played a tune written by Donald, 'The Tiree Association Centenary March', another written in honour of my Dad, titled simply 'Donald Campbell', and a lament I wrote myself, which I adapt each time I play it.

Creativity. I wrote a blog.

Curiosity. I read in the afternoon.

Diet. I ate well all day – no sweets, no chocolate, no booze.

Sleep. Afternoon nap.

Scenery. We were in one of the most beautiful parts of the world so I just sat for an hour and stared at Ben Nevis across the water.

Medication. I took it.

David S. I called him. He said I would be fine.

And I was.

*

Since becoming a writer, broadcaster and campaigner on mental health, I get letters and emails, and approaches in the street or on trains and buses and planes, from people who talk to me like I am their doctor. 'What should I do about my dad? He just won't get out of bed in the morning.' 'I am worried my sister is on the wrong medication, what do you advise me to do?' 'I have OCD – shall I tell my boss?' I have found myself resorting to a line that at least makes them laugh, usually, but also makes the point about my own limitations. 'I'm a spin doctor not a real doctor. You need to see a real doctor.'

My personal journey to get to the roots of my depression through psychiatry continues. But I have also learned along the way, as I now tell these 'patients', as Fiona and I call them, that there is a good deal else we can do for ourselves. As someone who doesn't believe that there's a higher power looking out for us, I've found that very valuable. Getting a handle on my depression, getting to know my enemy, has made me feel more in control of my fight with it. Of all the research I have done on the scientific side of things, a lot was fascinating and some useful, such as the strategy I now use for dealing with my guilt about Donald, which I came to in the MRI scanner. But the simple insight Dr Austin gave me with her jam jar visual is what has had the biggest impact on me and it has really resonated with many others I have talked to. A woman I met at a party told me she had chronic depression and anxiety, and a month later sent me a message I treasure:

'Your jam jar chat has helped me more than any of the pills.'

I am not entirely sure why this idea resonated with me so strongly. Partly – back to the theme of relationships, and the importance of the messenger – it was because Dr Austin was so enthusiastic, clear and compelling in how she explained the concept. It was also the simplicity, and I have been struck by how many others, on hearing me talk about it, have taken to the idea of the jam jar and created their own. Head teachers have sent me presentations they have done for the children in their charge. Employers I have spoken to do jam jar exercises with staff. At a mental health trust in Surrey, where I spoke to staff, they ended the day by designing their own jam jars, and sharing them. There is something in it that is very accessible: very quickly people can see the point that it is a straightforward device we can use to help ourselves. Being depressed is a kind of paralysis and the jam jar offers a way to take charge of your life again and build a way out of it, small step by step. And if you have never known depression, it is in any event a good way of thinking through the things that give your life meaning, purpose, pleasure and happiness.

I think this approach is all the more important when, as now, we have politicians who talk the talk on mental health, but under three successive Prime Ministers have failed to walk the walk. Though the debate on mental health is going in the right direction, a decade of austerity means services are not.

When Jeremy Hunt was Health Secretary, he called me in for a chat on mental health. He picked my brains. I picked his. Then he said something that left me open-mouthed. He said he had been watching a documentary about me in which I talked about my depression. 'I said to my wife, "why would Alastair Campbell get depression? He has a great life."' Open-mouthed. It is one thing for Joe Public to think depression is a lifestyle choice rather than an illness. This was the Health Secretary, the person in charge of the NHS.

When David Cameron was Prime Minister, he made a series of 'historic pledges'. One was that if you had psychosis you would see a psychiatrist within a maximum of two weeks. I have had psychosis. The physical health equivalent is being in a bad car crash, smashing through the windscreen and breaking a dozen bones as you bounce down the highway. No parity between mental and physical health there. 'Don't worry,' the ambulance driver tells the car crash victim lying bleeding in the road, 'we will have someone here for you in two weeks.'

When Theresa May spoke for the first time as Prime Minister outside Number 10, promising to address burning injustices, she claimed mental illness was one of them, and dealing with it would be her 'priority'. But 'priority' means 'more important than other things'. Brexit anyone? The words were easy. The injustices still burn. Many services have gone backwards. Child and adolescent mental health services, in many parts of the country, are in crisis.

I fear things will be even worse under a Prime Minister as reckless as Boris Johnson, who has never to my knowledge shown much interest in or understanding of mental health issues.

If the politicians won't deliver as they should, whether we like it or not we are going to have to take a lot more responsibility ourselves for our own mental health.

I think that trying to get good out of bad is a very human reaction. I have been struck, for example, in the work I do with the Time to Change campaign, the ambassadorships I have for Mind and Rethink, and my patronage of the Maytree Sanctuary for the Suicidal how many City banks and other big firms are starting to take mental health and mental illness seriously. For one thing, not to do so is bad for business. Most, including the Stock Exchange itself, have had experience of suicide during the financial crash. That experience has made them more aware not just of the tragedy and the waste, but the cost to them of losing expensive human assets, who need to be replaced. I am not saying that is their only motivation, but it is a part of it, justifiably so.

What I love about Time to Change is that it really is focused on changing people's attitudes, but understands this can have a broader, deeper impact. In the work I do for these charities, I often find myself telling the story of when my Mum gathered us around the kitchen table in Keighley – I was seven or eight – and told us our neighbour had cancer, adding: 'You mustn't tell anyone.' That was the culture of the time. Indeed, we used to call cancer 'the big C', such was the fear of the real thing. Now we all know what to say when a friend or relative has cancer, or when someone gets on a train, sits down opposite you, and takes off their hat to reveal mid-chemo baldness.

As a society we have developed the language so that we can understand, support and sympathise, make it easier for cancer charities to raise funds, and woe betide a government or NHS trust that dares to cut cancer care. Now we need to do the same for mental illness. It's time to break down the last great taboo, so that people are as open about their mental health as they are about their physical health, and feel neither shame nor fear in being so. I want us to become a society where we would no more tolerate seriously mentally ill people sleeping on the streets – as we do, in increasing numbers, all over the country – than we would walk past someone who fell off the pavement and broke an ankle, or who collapsed with a stroke or heart attack, without immediately trying to help. I could have hidden away my depression, my psychosis, my addictions, and followed Mum's desire that I should avoid any more scrutiny of my life. I know she was motivated by nothing more than love of me, and love of Donald. But I want – and I think there is a part of me that *needs* – to bear witness and I hope it will give others the desire, the courage if that is what is needed, to do the same.

Writing this book, and the work I do with mental health charities, is about fulfilment; about taking the bad and turning it into something good, a more creative expression of an experience and a time when I thought I was going to die.

I know I will never be entirely free of depression. I think anyone who's looking just to make their depression go away is unrealistic. The best I have been able to do is learn ways to make it easier to deal with. But, as they have really helped me, I am hoping that some of the techniques and ideas in this book might help others too, not just those who have depression, and those who worry they might, but those like Fiona, Rory, Calum and Grace who have to live with it in others.

The key lesson I have learned from the many depressives, their families and friends, and healthcare professionals I have met over the years is the importance of sharing your story, being honest both with yourself and with other people and talking honestly about your feelings – because however lonely you might feel, you don't have to be alone. And no matter how low you get, no matter how close to ten, there is a way back. I'm still here, and even on the darkest days it is better to be alive than dead.

David Sturgeon was so right.

AC: What is the fucking point, David?
DS: The point of what?
AC: Life.
DS: The point of life is to live it.

I might as well get on with it. I hope you do too.

AFTERWORD: HOW TO LIVE WITH DEPRESSION (WHEN IT'S NOT YOUR OWN)

Fiona Millar

'What is it like living with Alastair Campbell?' I get asked this a lot and my answer, not entirely in jest, is usually 'Bloody difficult . . . but never boring'. From the moment we met almost forty years ago, it was clear that Alastair was a complex, charismatic and challenging person. Anyone who has now read this book will be able to see that.

The first thing I noticed about him was his height and that he seemed rather conservative. He was wearing a sports jacket, shirt and tie, aged twenty-two, for heaven's sake, which felt pretty staid to someone like me, straight from unconventional 1970s North London via a year in California. Nevertheless, it quickly became clear that he was very different from everyone else I'd met – fiercely intelligent, exceptionally driven and with an outstanding ability for commanding the space around him and getting what he wanted. It was only later that I came to realise these high control needs, the constant urge to influence and make a difference, were an essential part of keeping himself on an even psychological keel.

Thrown together as trainee journalists on the *Mirror Group*'s scheme in the West of England, we started going out very quickly, probably moving in together much earlier than might have been the case if we hadn't been assigned to the same local paper in Tavistock, a sleepy West Devon market town. It was the start of a relationship that has lasted decades, given us three wonderful children and provided many highs but also some anguished lows, largely due to Alastair's undiagnosed depression and subsequent mental health roller coaster ride.

Tavistock in those days didn't offer many social options so our evenings out were generally spent in the pub. Looking back, and knowing what I know now, the levels of drinking in those early days ought to have rung loud alarm bells. Alastair had the capacity to devour huge amounts of alcohol while rarely appearing drunk or even hung over, and also able to churn out a phenomenal amount of copy. He was hugely ambitious and quickly made his mark in the town as a general reporter and sports columnist. As I could drive and had a car, I got the job of covering the much less glamorous parish councils and local women's institutes, and it was hard to keep up. Much more recently, writing a book about winning, he discovered the term 'maladaptive competitiveness', meaning that the desire to win or achieve an objective risks obscuring all else. He has it, I don't. My relative lack of competitive spirit, however, was probably a perfect match for his driven personality. To this day he is keen to exclaim 'I won' if he has slept longer, walked further, swum longer in the freezing outdoor pool we frequent, or the dog has run to him rather than me.

It was only later that I came to understand how some people use substances to manage the depression and anxiety, which are so often the flip side of high-functioning, competitive workaholism. Looking back at that younger me, and thinking of the advice I might give anyone who finds themselves in the same situation, my first tip would be to try to understand why your partner might be overusing or abusing drink or drugs.

This pressure, allied with frantic socialising, only got worse once we moved back to London and very quickly landed jobs on national papers as reporters, then political correspondents, by our mid-twenties. Nearly everyone, it felt, drank to what we now know is excess in 1980s Fleet Street. In Alastair's case this continued to mask his growing and serious mental health issues which exploded into the open in the mid-1980s when a change of job, followed by a period of intense stress, saw his drinking reach epic proportions.

His behaviour became increasingly erratic, irrational and aggressive. I remember at one point my Scottish father, who adored my charismatic, northern, bagpipe-playing, football-loving, suit-wearing boyfriend (and was adored in return as a drinking buddy as well as an in-law), taking me to one side and asking seriously: 'Are you sure you want to stay with him?' Even though my answer was an emphatic yes – I never really had a doubt – within weeks we had separated. Alastair moved into a hotel; radio silence descended between us until I got a 1.00 a.m. call to say he had been arrested and was in a police cell in Scotland.

I was shocked, of course, but not wholly surprised. It had been evident for some time that something was going badly wrong. As I flew to Scotland, I was anxious about what I might find there. My father came along for moral support and I needed it. When I walked into the ward I was faced with something I had never seen before, someone I thought I knew well but in a detached, vacant state, barely connecting with us. I remember feeling hugely protective of him and being terrified of reacting in the wrong way.

It felt a strange twist of fate that this hospital should be in Paisley, the town where my father had grown up and where we had spent many childhood holidays. I spent the days in the hospital and the evenings in my hotel room, where I alternated between floods of tears and desperate phone calls trying to find out how I could help him get better. This marked the start of phase two of our life together and it felt as though we were moving into a very dark, unknown future.

Alastair's breakdown was a seismic event and I have tried to relive that period many times since, trying to understand how and if it could have been avoided. I wish I had understood more about what 'mental health' meant. Before his breakdown there were many signs that I chose to ignore. Even then the cracks became most apparent on holiday. A photo from a trip to pre-glasnost Russia is still stuck to our fridge, showing Alastair downing a bottle of lemon vodka – for breakfast. It was clear that Alastair's obsessions with left versus right and the colours red and blue were becoming irrational. He would notice signs pointing to the left and right, or containing the colours red and blue, then invest them with mystical and unsettling significance.

Not long after this, he phoned me from a Fleet Street drinking den called Vagabonds claiming the landlord was sizing him up for a coffin, followed by his usual flat denials of my concerns that he might be ill. But this time I was so worried that I phoned his then boss on the fledgling and experimental *Today* newspaper to suggest he was seriously unwell and that together we should intervene, only to have my concerns dismissed and to be made to feel a complete fool both by him, and subsequently by Alastair. This exacerbated the ongoing trend in our relationship at times of crisis, a debilitating feeling of powerlessness and the assumption that there was something wrong with me, not him, if I were to question or challenge his behaviour or habits. I like to think that today, with more awareness of mental health, my younger self would be taken more seriously and would be more confident and self-assertive about seeking help.

It was only once Alastair had come through the worst of the crisis, after a short period on sedatives and anti-depressants and having convinced himself that drink was the cause of his breakdown, that the hard work really began. Restarting his career from the bottom was painful. A lot of people had thoroughly enjoyed the rapid fall from grace of the young Fleet Street high-flyer, and elaborate, false rumours shot round the Street about what had 'really' happened at the time of his arrest. It quickly became apparent who our real friends were, which taught me a lasting lesson about what true friendship is. He has his FFF – Fiona, family and friends – as the biggest part of his jam jar, and I have AFF – Alastair, family and friends. We are as close today as we have ever been.

More troubling in hindsight was his determination to get well without professional help. Alastair quit the booze, shunned psychiatrists, rebuffed Alcoholics Anonymous – a mistake thankfully not repeated by our son Calum many years later – and made a noisy virtue of curing himself. Initially that appeared to be entirely successful. He went on to be political editor of the *Daily Mirror*, was pivotal in the election of New Labour and commanded the political heights as Tony Blair's Director of Communications in Downing Street, where we both worked for six years. What wasn't as clear to me, and even less so to the outside world, was that in spite of his 'cure' he was still a high-functioning depressive and was probably ill throughout much of that period.

While we were all busy congratulating Alastair on his self-cure, we normalised and misread the workaholism and demonic energy, the mind-numbing crashes which would sometimes leave him unable to get out of bed at weekends, though I noticed bitterly that he would rouse himself to get to work on weekdays. This had a heavy impact both on our relationship and our young family. His moods, as you will have seen, are extreme.

Alastair is loyal, generous and very funny – he still makes me laugh more than anyone else. He is brilliant and selfless in a crisis and can be very kind, especially to friends in need, but his behaviour can also tip into something more dangerous. Once he sets his mind on an objective he cannot be budged from it; you can see why presidents and prime ministers would want him on their side but it isn't always healthy or pleasant to be around.

It took me too long to realise the incredibly complex nature of addictive, compulsive personalities and the impact of their behaviour on others. Now these incidents are ancient history and we can laugh at them. But they were horrible at the time.

Take, for example, the episode at a French service station where I went off to get him some lunch, but when I brought him back a ham baguette, he exploded at me. This wasn't what he wanted! Why didn't I know he hated ham? I didn't know because until then he hadn't. In fact when we first met the only sign of domestication in his lonely Plymouth bedsit had been a packet of ham and some bread rolls. But I know now that this banal detail is irrelevant. Something had triggered a meltdown that day on the motorway; the ham was an excuse, and the fact that he consequently refused to speak to me for at least three days at the start of a holiday with two young children really wasn't funny, and turned a period of our usually happy life together toxic. As usual I took the blame. Today I would probably laugh it off. I believe that form of depressive sulking probably stems from a need to control, and the quickest way to diffuse it is to expose it confidently using humour.

I suspect that much of this misery could have been avoided if Alastair had sought, immediately after his discharge from hospital, the professional help that he only acknowledged was necessary twenty years later. While he had had a bad experience with his first trip to the Maudsley, I think he was probably looking for an excuse to go it alone, to 'look after myself'. I had never heard the story of his childhood fight in the Hebrides until now, but his reaction, to turn inwards and rely on himself, does not surprise me at all.

This would be my second tip to the younger me, and to others today. If you are in any doubt about the mental health of someone you love, fight as hard as you can to cajole them into seeking and finding help. This is hard to do without making an already volatile person feel additionally pressured – that dread word 'nagging' comes to mind (more blame). Without wanting to sound like a stuck record, it is about trying not to allow their mood to distort your own, and dispassionately to set out constructive routes out of the gloom. It is about helping them reach the point of understanding that they need help, not assuming they can see things as clearly and as rationally as you do.

So, it took another couple of decades to realise that the start of a holiday often marks a flashpoint for Alastair. Unmoored from the containing pressure of work, being busy and changing the world, the prospect of days of looming emptiness ahead (something many people might relish) often triggers anxiety, depression and lashing out, followed probably by a healthy dose of guilt and self-hate. Alastair can work more hours on holiday than most people work in a normal week. Indeed, much of this book was written at a kitchen table in France. And his manic drive accompanied us to dinner one night at a local restaurant where Alastair, who lists 'bad service in restaurants' among his obsessions, became so infuriated by the slowness of our waitress that he began clearing tables himself. Difficult . . . but never boring.

Knowledge is power, and since we have come to understand the pressure of that transition to relaxation, mainly through spending more time in France together in the last ten years since the children left school, it has become easier to manage. Mind you, only a few months ago Grace and I were there alone, chilling out, waiting for Alastair to arrive a bit later from a round of work, charity and public-speaking engagements abroad.

Somewhat guiltily, we found ourselves slightly dreading his arrival because we knew our tranquil routine of yoga, box set and autumnal walks would soon be shattered by a deluge of noisy activity, as it duly was: 'Why am I here, I should be at home fighting Brexit?'; 'Is this all you do all day?'; 'Yoga is ruining the world' (a recent favourite); 'Have you two finally retired?' And all before lunch. It passes now more quickly than it did and, mercifully, the kind of suicidal low he describes experiencing in Scotland is rare.

Then there were my own feelings of guilt and failure for being unable to make him happy at times when his depression is really setting in or at feeling excluded when his mania is taking over. This has left me sad, for though I have experienced grief, I have never known depression. Even now I find it impossible to comprehend what it must feel like to be so preoccupied with changing the world that loved ones barely get a look in. Sir Alex Ferguson once advised Alastair to see an election campaign as a tunnel into which only the essential people were allowed. I often felt that I wasn't on that list. But I cannot imagine either how it must feel to be so depressed that getting out of bed is a struggle, although in our case it was never as straightforward as that.

It was a hurtful puzzle that Alastair could get up for work and function seemingly normally, be affectionate and engaged with the children but reserve his silent, black-dog moods for me. I still don't fully understand this, and he can't explain it other than to say he was sending the signal that he wants me to be there while not actually wanting me to be there, or that I am the only person to whom he will expose his full vulnerabilities. But I now accept this without allowing myself to take the emotionally draining blame which inevitably used to follow, even if it means consciously telling myself over and over that it *is* about him, not me. Over the years I have spent a lot of time venting my anger and misery by pounding up and down the lanes of my local swimming pool. I swim every day and the physical release it offers has helped me so much. I can't recommend regular exercise enough.

Not enough is said about the partners of people who are mentally ill, but whenever I have spoken publicly about our life together, and made this point about the partner feeling guilty, I have been inundated with messages from people in the same situation, grateful that I have articulated their own experiences. After we left Downing Street, and there was more time to reflect without the distraction of a high-octane day job, his crashes became longer and more frequent, culminating in the episode on Hampstead Heath when fear, anger, helplessness, loss of purpose, self-loathing – I will never know which – caused Alastair to start punching himself in the face. It was only when Philip Gould urged Alastair to see a psychiatrist, David Sturgeon, who helped both of us understand more about his illness and led Alastair to accept the need for regular therapy and medication, that things finally started to improve. It also helped me to understand my own emotions, and the part I may have played in the difficult times, how to ride out the low points and above all not to see his depression as being about me. In particular, I remember David explaining to me that Alastair's high need for control effectively meant that at times he saw me as an extension of himself, almost like an extra limb, and if he couldn't get me to behave the way he wanted, it caused him real pain.

Also enormously helpful were two slim books, *The Addictive Personality* by Craig Nakken, and *On Forgiveness* by Richard Holloway, which David asked us to read. Both explained so much to me about the impact addicts can have on other people and about how letting go of anger and blame can be liberating rather than scary. If this intervention had happened twenty years earlier, I wonder how different our lives might have been?

Alastair now sees my over-reliance on his getting professional help when he is feeling very bad as indicating a worrying degree of helplessness on my part, but it is in fact a perfect description of how I have often felt over the last forty years. It is true that whenever he is on a plunge, my first instinct is to ask why it is happening (I've yet to receive a good answer) and the second is to suggest he goes to see David. It is interesting that Alastair uses exactly the same word – helpless – to describe how he feels when a sudden plunge is upon him.

*

I know people who feel they couldn't stay with partners once serious mental health issues threaten their own wellbeing. Several have contacted me to tell me their stories over the years, but I can honestly say that I have never seriously considered leaving Alastair. About fifteen years ago I wrote an article for *The Times*, to coincide with the release of his diaries, about our life together. It included one line which has, needless to say, been thrown back at me more than once, mostly humorously, over the years. '*On balance* I am glad we stayed together,' I wrote.

'Oh wow,' he said at the time. 'Not love him to bits ... this man of my dreams ... but on balance it is just about OK being with him?' I would go further today. We are much happier now, more tolerant and understanding of each other and his illness, and the impact it has on our relationship. But it would be dishonest to say there haven't been a few moments when I questioned if it was right to stay. I am a loyal person. We both had parents who had long happy marriages and I wanted our children to have that stability (without the marriage bit). My default position has always been to want to help Alastair get better, even if that might get rebuffed or feels pointless. But I have learned to accept my own limitations in this, and to understand that unless someone actually wants help, you can't make them take it.

Thanks to good psychiatric support, the right medication and increased self-awareness on both our parts, I would say our lives are better than ever. We have various separate interests now, and maybe it wasn't the best idea for us to live and work together for long periods both as journalists and in politics. I don't go to Burnley, for example, where Alastair spends so many Saturdays in the football season that he jokes that he has a completely separate life there. But I know that the best thing for his mental health sometimes is to be on the move, letting off steam elsewhere. His riposte to my 'difficult but never boring' joke is that I am 'boring but never difficult', but maybe that is because we complement each other in a way that means, fingers crossed, though happily unmarried, we will beat our parents' records.

Like his mother, I had concerns when Alastair first started talking openly about his mental health. I could see his motivation – it has proved to be another route for him to be busy and instigate change – but I worried about our privacy. I was wrong. We are now stopped by people – in the street, on Hampstead Heath and at the swimming pool – who want to talk more about their own, or a loved one's, mental health than the state of our politics. Reading his book, and its attempt to explain one person's experience of depression and uncover potential cures, has been another step on that journey of understanding for me. I thought I knew him inside out, but I have found things out about Alastair that surprised me in these pages. I feel I understand him even better now. I hope the growing awareness of mental illness, the willingness of public figures to talk openly about their struggles and the media coverage will help other people.

So much would have been different thirty years ago, when Alastair was heading towards his nervous breakdown, if I had been aware of a fraction of the information and advice that is now in the public domain about this far too well-hidden illness. These are challenging times for people seeking psychiatric support on the NHS, but if I did get the chance to advise my twenty-something self I would say get professional help as soon as possible; be there for the people you love in a non-judgemental way; find something you can do for yourself to relieve the stress; and above all, avoid blaming yourself. The chances are you are not to blame for this.

With the right support, mental health conditions can be managed and alleviated. It will never be plain sailing but I hope the unvarnished story of our family's experience gives others courage and the confidence that they can come through. It is better to live, and live well. Even during his less frequent low points today, I now know that is possible.

When Alastair looks back on the intense, difficult years he spent at the heart of politics, working with Tony Blair and then Gordon Brown, he says that 'on balance', knowing all that was to come and its costs, it was all worth it and he would do it again. Looking back on our decades-long relationship and its great ups and terrible downs, I think I would say the same. While there are still moments of pain and frustration in our relationship, I know enough to realise they will probably always be there but now I also know that they will pass. I can't imagine life without Alastair.

And how is this for progress? Alastair has let me have the final word. I doubt very much that would have happened back in the early 1980s, in the trainees' Portakabin in Plymouth, where our emotional roller coaster of a relationship first began.

POSTSCRIPT*

On a lovely sunny morning in mid-May, I am settling down to write something I wish I didn't have to write. Oh Lord, that sounds like the start of a suicide note, which is hardly the best ending to a book on depression, especially one that I want you to find uplifting and helpful. I wrote this book in one world, you're reading it in another. I wish that meant that *Living Better* was now unnecessary, and everything it covers nothing more than an interesting historical footnote. Sadly, however, that is far from the case. We were already facing something of a mental health crisis before coronavirus. Covid-19 has made matters a whole lot worse.

It is now two months since I went into my own lockdown, well ahead of official advice and amid some pretty cack-handed government dithering. I could see the signs. We all could – even if Boris Johnson and his hapless crew were still desperately trying to ignore them as he holidayed and they celebrated 'getting

* Sorry for taking back the last word, Fiona.

Brexit done'. The news became increasingly grim: from China, to Iran, to Italy, the virus was showing no respect for national boundaries or politicians' bluster. As a life-long asthmatic, with two brothers dead in part because of respiratory issues, I had seen and heard enough to know it was time to take care and stay at home.

So, since Sport Relief in Manchester on Friday, 13 March, my house and Hampstead Heath for a morning walk are pretty much the only places I have seen. I am not great at any kind of isolation to be frank. I don't mind my own company, but I enjoy it best when I am travelling, working in new environments, doing new things. There is not much of that available within my own four walls, and with every speaking engagement in my diary cancelled.

Initially there was a strange novelty to life in lock-down. I felt faintly and inappropriately superior for having made the decision myself, guided by the science dare I say, rather than waiting for the Cabinet clowns. Also, things felt safer inside my house even when, outside, it looked as if the world was, quite literally, falling apart. During the day it was mostly OK, but I began to find it increasingly hard to sleep. Despite all my efforts to self-police – eat sensibly, avoid alcohol, go to bed early – my waking time seemed to get earlier and earlier, with 3.55 a.m. the earliest and 5 a.m. the average.

Every morning it was still dark as I tried not to disturb Fiona as she slept, and I crept downstairs to plonk myself on the sofa and find out what was happening across the world. In the early days, I tried to give the government the benefit of the doubt. But after a while, I couldn't hold back. I knew all too well what it was like to be inside Number 10 as a crisis unfolded, and that knowledge and experience added an unsettling extra dimension to every briefing, interview or media conference. It was not a comforting time to be able to read between the lines. I sensed that not just I, but everyone, was feeling the same kind of powerlessness a depressive knows all too well, as the depression works its way into every aspect of your mind and body. Now Covid-19 was having that same effect on everyone too, all of us trapped in our own bubbles, looking on helplessly as things were going from bad to worse.

It doesn't help in these circumstances that people seem to think I know what is going on and can do something about it. A flood of emails from friends and colleagues asked what I thought was happening and what my advice would be. I watched as other leaders, notably Andrew Cuomo in New York and Jacinda Ardern in New Zealand, identified the potential mental health consequences of the crisis early on, at a time when our government was still not remotely on top of the immediate crisis, let alone the medium- and long-term implications. Nor were my reflections on what would be required helped by considering that Johnson had appointed Nadine Dorries as minister for mental health.

I did my best to make myself very busy. Looking through the sheer volume of words I was writing most days (they are all stored on my website, under 'lockdown rants, rambles and ruminations'), I was clearly becoming more than a bit manic. Fiona thought so too. She has had to live with my ups and downs much longer than anyone else, and is best at spotting the signs. I can be very good fun to be with at the manic end of the scale, but it can also be wearing; and it always leads to a crash, eventually.

The questions then are how long, and how deep?

When happy, I have a very strange habit of serenading Fiona to the tune of Scotland's national anthem 'Flower of Scotland', and making up new words as I go, according to where we are and what we are doing. So, first thing in the morning, in the bathroom, something like this:

> *Oh power of sertraline,*
> *What would I do,*
> *Without my pills?*
> *I'm taking them right now,*
> *To keep my head on the straight,*
> *And fucking narrow,*
> *Another day beckons,*
> *How lucky are we both,*
> *To be alive?*

I can sing that tune, and apply new words to any situation I'm in, on tap. Sometimes it makes Fiona laugh. Sometimes it makes her worry. She definitely knows it is a warning sign when I've got one verse for the bathroom, then another verse for the stairs:

> *Oh flower of staircase,*
> *How many steps*
> *Must you descend?*
> *Till reaching the kitchen*
> *To make a coffee for me*

> *And then some porridge*
> *With toppings aplenty*
> *To take the taste away*
> *From boring oats.*

Then another verse when the porridge arrives:

> *Oh flower of porridge,*
> *What shall we put,*
> *Upon you now?*
> *Banana or honey?*
> *Or eat you just as you are?*
> *Then get our boots on,*
> *And go for a walk with*
> *Our wonderful dog called Skye*
> *Who gives us joy.*

You're getting the picture. But then suddenly I woke one morning, and there was no singing, no messing around, and what an old university friend used to call my 'demonic energy' had gone. Fiona has always asked what triggers a plunge and I never really know. It might have been the lockdown. It might have been that for all the thousands of words I had written about ways in which the government could improve their handling of the crisis, it was probably not making a blind bit of difference. It might have been that my publisher and agent had finally persuaded me that I should move the publication of this book from May to September. It might have been related to the fact that in the week it happened, on consecutive days my Mum would have been ninety-six and my Dad ninety-eight.

The silly songs and the hyperactive writing had not been the only signs. Poor sleep is always a danger signal and I had had weeks of it.

So one day, even though I slept through past 6 a.m. for the first time in ages, I woke feeling empty, my head foggy; not with the truly deadening feeling that comes with a major depression, but the pangs – the beginnings of it.

The next day, I awarded the gold medal in the 'Tree of the Day' contest I had invented, to amuse myself and my social media followers, to a tree that was dead, flat on its back, a bit ugly. The silver and bronze medallists looked as though they had stopped giving a toss how they come over to the outside world. Day two was worse than day one, and day three was worse than day two. Fiona and I both worried the downward spiral was upon me. The danger signs were strong and in the old days that might have been it, but now I know how to arrest it.

Now I can recognise the symptoms, I know how to start dealing with the illness before it overwhelms me. Based on my own experience of depression and its flip-side, anxiety, I started drawing up a list of twenty things that I had found helpful in lockdown. Like this book, my list takes a very personal approach to dealing with depression. I have discovered through trial and error that what works for me is filling my jam jar, one positive thing at a time, stone by stone. My experience of depression does not make me an expert in the illness; it just makes me an expert in mine. Everyone will be different, so some of these ideas may not work for you. But I hope that within them, there might be something for all.

When I published the list on my blog and on Twitter, it really seemed to strike a chord and was picked up by newspapers, magazines, companies and charities in different parts of the world. It led to old friends in Switzerland, South Africa and Australia getting in touch. Here is an updated version of it, because I think there are some interesting lessons from lockdown, with all the distractions of our everyday lives stripped away. Writing it helped me, and I hope reading it will help you too:

1. **Try to stay active**. When your mood is low, your energy is low. The temptation to do nothing is strong. Try to resist it.

2. **Exercise.** Low mood means low energy. Trapped in the house, the temptation to do nothing is strong. Try to resist it. It is very easy to think, 'Ah well, I can't go out, so I'll sit and watch telly all day, and raid the fridge and the cupboard every half-hour.' There is so much capacity for exercise, even in the home. Walking/running up and down stairs. Press ups, squats, star jumps and running on the spot don't require lots of space.

3. **Watch your diet.** See the 'raid the fridge' point in 2. Try to eat as healthily as possible. For many people, boredom = eat; dislocation = eat; loneliness = eat. It's important to be aware of it, maybe keep a food diary in which you record what you eat, share it with someone doing the same thing and swap ideas.

4. **Watch the booze.** Someone tweeted about lockdown, 'This is like Christmas without the fun!' I

think we all know what he means. And most know the temptation to drink more at Christmas, or on holiday. It's best to resist. Try to drink less than you were, not more.

5. **Sleep.** Very, very important. I know I have not been practising what I preach here. But it is partly because I have insomniac nights occasionally that I am so focused on the need to sleep well.

6. **Read books not newspapers.** I think it is important not to overconsume media at a time like this. Books that have nothing to do with the current crisis, fiction or non-fiction, can be such a wonderful release.

7. **Cut down on social media.** Again, there is so much happening, things are moving so fast, and it is natural to want to try to stay on top of events. But endlessly scrolling through social media feeds is not the best way to do it.

8. **Listen to music regularly.** Very much better for you than the radio or the telly! I have been listening to Brel and Elvis, Piaf and Abba when on the exercise bike.

9. Even better – **make music**! I alerted my neighbours that my regular bagpipe playing would become a lot more regular and I would be trying out new tunes. There is no doubt that playing and listening to music has helped me keep on a reasonably even keel, mentally, most of the time. And to Mr Jonathan Wheeler of Birstall, Leicestershire, who wrote to the *Guardian* asking if I was playing the pipes 'to make music or to enforce social distancing', I say three things through the smile he inspired: 1. Bugger off. 2. Those

who don't like bagpipes have never heard them played well – or never listened properly. 3. My neighbours complain when I don't play, not when I do!

10. **'Think in ink.'** I bet you can't guess who said that. It was Marilyn Monroe. And it is one of my life rules. That's obvious, you might think, since I am a writer. But thinking in ink can help us all, whether or not you plan to publish what you write. Why are lists so helpful/common? Because we think in ink. Why do so many people write diaries and journals? Because there is a therapeutic benefit to committing thoughts to paper.

11. (I suppose number 1 ought to be the most important point, but actually this one is.) **Really look after the people closest to you.** Be as nice and as kind as you can possibly be. I am very lucky in that if I was only allowed one person to be locked away with twenty-four hours a day, it would be Fiona (and most of the time she feels the same about me). But I dread to think what it would be like to be living through this with a partner or a family you don't want to be with, let alone to be in a relationship of abuse and violence. Each day I am trying to do something that I don't normally do, to make sure Fiona knows I know how lucky I am. That can be anything from telling her that I know how lucky I am to – wait for it – unloading the dishwasher in the morning. Yes, I did, albeit at 4.45 a.m.

12. **Keep in touch with the people you would normally be in touch with.**

13. **Get in touch with someone you've lost contact with.**
14. **Do something good for someone else every day.**
15. **If you are finding it hard to do difficult things, try a few easy ones first.** When I am depressed, and I know my mood and energy is going to be low, in my mind I make a big deal of little things. I challenge myself to brush my teeth, and when I have done it, I tell myself how well I did. I tell myself that shaving is a hard thing to do, and when I've done it, I feel better. If I can turn the radio on, I can turn my mind on.
16. **Stay curious.** This is related to points 6, 8 and 10. This really is a time to expand knowledge and try new things. My birthday came during lockdown. (Fiona gave me a Goethe Institut online German course to brush up my once-fluent German. I now sing German lyrics to her, to the tune of 'Oh Blumen von Schottland.')
17. **Enjoy nature, in or out.** If you're stuck inside, watch nature documentaries. If you follow me on social media you will know I have been posting 'Tree of the Day' photos. I cannot tell you how much pleasure I have got, on our morning walk with the dog, from deciding which tree to pick. It is especially wonderful right now as the birds are starting to sing more.
18. **Remember that all crises end eventually.** All good things come to an end, and so do all bad things. Clearly, by the time this one is over, there will have been a lot of death, a lot of grief, a lot of suffering. But it will end, and most of the world will still be here. That is not a bad thought to cling to. So . . .

19. **Keep things in perspective.** Don't panic. And finally . . .
20. **See an opportunity in every setback**. The whole world is going to have to take this approach when the crisis is over, but we can all do it in our own lives now. Get good out of bad.

So here we are, mid-May. My rage at the incompetence and venality of Boris Johnson and his team shows no sign of abating. My frustration at being unable to travel grows too. But for most of the time I have been enjoying lockdown much more than I thought I would. The weather has been good, Fiona and I have not had a single serious row and our dog Skye has never been happier. She can't believe her luck to have us both at home so much.

There is a very long list of things I have missed in lockdown. I doubt you'll be surprised to hear that Burnley Football Club comes in at number 1. I have kept in touch with my friends there. Manager Sean Dyche tolerates my constant attempts to talk football with him; I tolerate his constant attempts to talk politics, or more accurately the crisis, with me. (He is among those who assume I might know what is happening inside Downing Street.) Number 2 on my 'things I miss' list is the Lido on Parliament Hill, my yearning for a swim growing each day as we walk past it at the entrance to the Heath. I miss long train journeys. I don't miss airports or planes, but I do miss the places they take me to.

I miss restaurants. I miss Pret. I miss live sport on TV (the re-runs of old games just haven't done it for me). I miss cinema, theatre and live music. I miss my Albanian barber Alex Palushi. Fiona has done an OK job, but my hair has been growing back very unevenly. I miss seeing friends and extended family. I miss real meetings with real people, in offices. I miss chats with random strangers. I miss people who come up and talk to me, on buses, trains, walking down the street. I especially miss the chats about mental health, when people just stop me and tell me their stories. It still happens a bit when walking the dog, and one day on the Heath recently we had a wonderful, though very sad, chat with a woman who had lost her brother to suicide some years ago. But it happens far less frequently than when I am buzzing around the country, and of course people have understandably been keeping their distance.

And one thing I miss intensely is something that never happened – the reason I wish I wasn't writing this postscript at all. Today should have been a really good day. It's 14 May: the publication day of this book. The climax of a busy week, due to kick off with the *Observer* running extracts on Sunday; last night a charity event to talk about the book; tonight a literary festival; and lots of interviews for press, radio, TV.

That was how it was meant to be. Then along came coronavirus. In the grand scheme of things, the postponement of a book does not, of course, merit the same angst as tens of thousands of deaths making the UK one of the worst-hit countries in the world, or the economic slide and consequent social tensions that Covid-19 is inflicting on the world. But it certainly underlines its impact, just one among many hundreds, thousands, millions, billions of changes in people's lives, large and small, that we have had to live with, and adapt to, since coronavirus replaced Brexit and football as the go-to subject of most of my conversations – and everyone else's.

So why was I so reluctant to call it off when the publisher first suggested we wait until it became clearer how the crisis would pan out, and see whether life might get back to some kind of normality?

Well, first, because I am not sure 'normality' as we understand it will be likely for a long time to come. Coronavirus has done something rarely achieved in these times of media proliferation, filter bubbles and echo chambers – it went from zero awareness to universal awareness (and impact) in a matter of weeks. It went to the top of the agenda of virtually every organisation in the world: governments, public services, businesses, councils, charities, sports clubs . . . Everybody has been affected in some way.

Having written the book, I wanted to get it out there and talk about it, hopefully make it a success, and use it further to shift the dial in the debate on mental health at a time when, amid all the other pressures on governments, I fear it will slip down the agenda again. The thought of delaying it added to my growing sense of being in limbo, and I worried about what that might do to me, mentally. The process of writing this book was one reason my mental health had been pretty robust recently, and I had been looking forward to getting out there and sharing what I have learned. I resisted and resisted, therefore, even as all the bookshops were shuttered, events were cancelled further and further into the future, and the media understandably fixated almost solely on coronavirus, until eventually I ran out of arguments against delaying and gave in. So here we are, with a September launch, and this new postscript being written in May.

My publisher wasn't just worried about the publication date – there was also the title. I hope you like *Living Better.* I like it. I am living better than I used to. And I hope that people who read this book, and perhaps adopt some of the thinking and the ideas in it, will live better too. It wasn't my first choice, however. Originally this book was called *Better to Live*, as in, better to live than to die. But also *Better to Live*, as in, 'here's how ... here's how I learned to live better and, who knows, maybe it will help you to live better too.' But day after day, as the death toll rose, this title seemed increasingly insensitive. Of course it is better to live, but so many didn't have that choice. How is someone going to feel, I wondered, maybe still in the throes of grief as they walk past a bookshop and notice the book in the window, or see me pop up on TV and say, you know what, it really is better to live? When several of the pro-Boris Johnson newspapers felt able to run huge headlines about 'Happy Monday' on what turned out to be false suggestions that the lockdown might be about to be lifted; on the day we actually overtook Italy in the European death league tables; the *Sun*, on a day when almost nine hundred people died, had a front-page headline 'Now that's a good Friday!' just because Johnson was out of intensive care. I wondered what on earth someone who had lost a loved one to this virus, so ineptly managed by the government, would have thought on seeing such gross insensitivity. So, *Living Better* it is.

It's my favourite of the books I have written so far, and it has my favourite cover. That's the work of talented young artist Naomi Edmondson who paints legal street art across Britain with the goal of 'promoting hope and optimism to bring a little light to people having a dark day'. (Here's her website if you want to find out more: survivaltechniques.co.uk)

My editor Georgina Laycock, in arguing for delay, said she felt more and more people might, as a direct result of the crisis, experience the kind of depression and anxiety I already know all too well, and that coronavirus and its impact would therefore make it more relevant, not less.

That may very well be right. The first item in my inbox when I woke up this morning was an email from my friend and fellow depressive Geoff Gallop, the former premier of Western Australia. He was forwarding a report by Professor Ian Hickie of the University of Sydney's Brain and Mind Centre, warning that suicide rates could rise by up to fifty per cent in the wake of the catastrophic and prolonged economic impact of Covid-19. The report argued that the best-case scenario was a twenty-five per cent increase in suicides in Australia, with the likelihood of about forty per cent of those being among young people. Professor Hickie said the modelling indicated that if the economy deteriorated further, the figure would escalate to a fifty per cent increase in the number of lives lost to suicide, with rural and regional areas hardest hit.

For Australia as a whole, this would mean between 750 and 1,500 additional deaths in the next year on top of the

3,000 suicide deaths that occur annually already, and he warned that those numbers are likely 'to persist for up to five years if the economic downturn lasts more than twelve months'. So that is Australia, which at the time of writing has had fewer than 7,000 cases and just ninety-seven deaths. What the eventual impact in the UK might be is anyone's guess, with deaths in the tens of thousands and the Bank of England forecasting the economy will shrink by fourteen per cent while unemployment doubles; it is not a happy situation. Not for nothing is the word for sustained economic slump . . . depression. It certainly seems inevitable that once we emerge from this crisis, we will do so accompanied by a veritable tsunami of psychological and psychiatric distress.

Parking economics for the moment, think of the mental health consequences for NHS staff who have been dealing with this; for the terrified, low-paid key workers who have kept our infrastructure going; for families unable to say farewell, console or bury loved ones; for parents trying to home school, work full time and pretend everything is all right; for children removed from their friends and trapped at home, the school year wiped out along with the exams they have studied for; for workers seeing their livelihoods vanish; for couples forced to confront unfixable cracks in their relationships; for older people learning that they have to be afraid of everyone. Most people, at some point, have felt anxious, paranoid and lonely. And with no physical contact to comfort them. No hugs or even handshakes. Social distancing may be necessary, but that doesn't make it good for anyone.

Perhaps those of us who are used to depression may have something of an advantage here, however. We who have known our troubled minds are used to things coming along and disturbing our equilibrium to its foundations. For many, this has been a new experience. More than once on my morning walk, and in recent emails and exchanges on social media, people have said to me that they have been beginning to 'understand what it must be like'.

My published diaries have often been described as 'intensely personal', and when first transcribing them I remember being shocked at just how often I seemed to be depressed. But in those days I was seeking to keep the depression at bay and escape it in any way that I could, not least through obsessive work. In writing this book I have been confronting it head-on in pursuit of better understanding, and I've found ways of living better with it.

In the midst of this darkness there is still much to be grateful for. And while the government has not shown much kindness, empathy or human understanding, that has often been counterbalanced by the warmth, kindness and sympathy of others. One of the features of lockdown I most enjoyed was everyone gathering on their doorsteps to clap and cheer for the NHS and care workers every Thursday night. Never one to do things by halves, I even wrote a special tune, 'Our Neighbours, Our Nurses', for the lovely nurse who lives next door and ceremonially piped her up the street as she came home from a double shift. I also want to thank all those people – the well-meaning ones, not the bots with lots of numbers after their social media names – who have asked me to take better care of myself, because I seem to be getting up too early to rant and rage at the world.

I have definitely had highs and lows during this time, as have so many others, but I really am doing fine.

Meanwhile, a Eurasian wren (I know this because I have a new songbird recognition app on my phone – 'Shazam for birds', Grace calls it) has just landed on my window ledge and is singing loudly. It looks and sounds happy, perhaps because birds no longer have to compete with planes for mastery of the skies. Fiona is downstairs in her office and we will meet up for lunch in a few hours. I have put on some Scottish folk music and I turn back to finish writing this. Skye has followed me upstairs and has settled down on the sofa, for yet another snooze. Life is not bad at all.

I know my depression will always be a part of me. I've accepted that now. I still have suicidal thoughts and dark days, and I always will. But at least now I can recognise them, I feel them coming on, and I can deal with them better than I used to. There may one day be a vaccine for Covid-19. But I doubt there will ever be a vaccine or a cure for depression. It is part of the human condition; it is certainly part of mine. I've spent decades learning to live with that. And now through trial and error, through medication and therapy, through highs and lows, above all through grief and love, I have finally got to know my enemy. I live better for having dealt with it. And I deal with it, through living better. I hope that for some of you out there, this book can help you do the same.

Alastair Campbell
14 May 2020

HELPFUL INFORMATION

In *Living Better* I've talked very much about my own experience and what has helped me to survive depression. The key word there is 'help,' and often it is about knowing what is out there, and knowing how to access it.

In addition to the NHS (treatment and support often good, but too often dependent on where you live, and all too often with long waits and staff under massive pressure) there are lots of organisations doing great work to help us feel and get better.

The following listing of helplines and websites (gathered with the help of my friends at Mind) is by no means complete, but it gives a good selection.

To talk about anything that is upsetting you, you can contact **Samaritans** 24 hours a day, 365 days a year. Call 116 123 (free from any phone), email jo@samaritans.org or visit some branches in person (check their website for details: samaritans. org). You can also call the Welsh language line on 0808 164 0123 (7 p.m.–11 p.m. every day).

If you're experiencing a mental health problem or supporting someone else in mental distress, you can call **SANEline** on 0300 304 7000 (4.30 p.m.–10.30 p.m. every day).

If you're under 25, you can call **The Mix** on 0808 808 4994 (Sunday–Friday 2 p.m.–11 p.m.), request support by email using the form on their website (themix.org.uk) or use their crisis text messenger service.

If you suffer from panic attacks, phobias or obsessive compulsive behaviours, you can call **No Panic** on 0844 967 4848; their youth helpline is 0330 606 1174.

If you're under 35 and struggling with suicidal feelings, or you're concerned about a young person who might be struggling, you can call **Papyrus HOPELINEUK** on 0800 068 4141 (weekdays 9 a.m.–10 p.m., weekends and bank holidays 2 p.m.–10 p.m.), email pat@papyrus-uk.org or text 07860 039967.

If you identify as male, you can call the **Campaign Against Living Miserably** (CALM) on 0800 58 58 58 (5 p.m.–midnight every day) or use their webchat service (see their website for details: thecalmzone.net).

If you're a student, you can look on the **Nightline** website to see if your university or college offers a night-time listening service. Nightline phone operators are all students too.

If you struggle with anxiety, call **Anxiety UK** on 03444 775 774 (weekdays 9.30 a.m.–5.30 p.m), text 07537 416 905 or email support@anxietyuk.org.

If you are feeling profoundly suicidal, The Maytree Sanctuary for the Suicidal provides short-term residential support to help through crisis. Call 020 7263 7070 or visit their site: maytree.org.uk.

If you identify as gay, lesbian, bisexual or transgender, and are struggling, you can call **Switchboard** on 0300 330 0630 (10 a.m.–10 p.m. every day), email chris@switchboard.lgbt or use their webchat service. Phone operators all identify as LGBT+.

If you live in Wales, you can call the **Community Advice and Listening Line** (C.A.L.L.) on 0800 132 737 (open 24/7) or text 'help' followed by a question to 81066.

In Scotland, you can call the **Scottish Association for Mental Health** (SAMH; samh.org.uk) on 0141 530 1000 or email enquire@samh.org.uk or contact **Support In Mind Scotland** (see their website for details: supportinmindscotland.org.uk).

For more options, visit the **Helplines Partnership** website (helplines.org) for a directory of UK helplines. **Mind's Infoline** (0300 123 3393 or text 86463) can also help you find services that can support you. If you're outside the UK, the **Befrienders Worldwide** website (befrienders.org) has a tool to search by country for emotional support helplines around the world.

HELPFUL INFORMATION

As well as phone numbers to call, some organisations routinely offer support in other ways – which could include emails, text messages or web chat.

Mind's website (mind.org.uk) is a fund of helpful information ranging from an A to Z of mental health to a supportive online community (for over 18s) elefriends.org.

Rethink Mental Illness are doing great work helping improve the quality of life of people with mental illness. Details of their advice and information service are at rethink.org.uk.

I have discussed my issues with addiction and there are various specific organisations that deal with addiction:

Adfam adfam.org.uk. Information and support for friends and family of people with drug or alcohol problems.

Alcoholics Anonymous (AA) alcoholics-anonymous.org.uk, tel. 0800 9177 650. Help and support for anyone with alcohol problems.

Beating Addictions beatingaddictions.co.uk. Information about a range of addictive behaviours and treatments.

FRANK talktofrank.com, tel. 0300 123 6600. Confidential advice and information about drugs, their effects and the law.

Gamblers Anonymous gamblersanonymous.org.uk. Support groups for anyone wanting to stop gambling.

Turning Point turning-point.co.uk. Provides health and social care services for people with drug, alcohol and mental health problems.

We Are With You wearewithyou.org.uk. Supports people with drug, alcohol or mental health problems, and also their friends and family.

BUILD YOUR OWN JAM JAR

So, if you have got this far, and if you are anything like many of the people I have told of this journey, you may well be thinking, 'I fancy making my own jam jar.'

Here is where you start.

The jam jar. Squat. Solid.

And in the bottom part is the sediment you will never be able to remove . . . your genes. (Draw them as circles.)

On top of them, there is your life, the good and the bad, the forgotten and the unforgettable, all mixing up (draw those elements as triangles) and sometimes getting dangerously close to overflowing, and the illness that comes with that.

To stave that off, create more space for life, and push back on the threat of your jam jar overflowing into illness, you can add your own extensions to the jam jar.

Mine started with FFF, **key relationships**. I suggest everyone starts there. Get the key relationships right and your jam jar grows.

Then **meaningful activity**. Your choice. For many this will be about work, but even if you do like what you do – and especially if you don't – we all need other interests that motivate, amuse and excite us.

But I think we all need the same fundamentals – sleep, nutrition, exercise. Eat well, sleep well and stay physically fit and you have three very large rings to grow your jam jar.

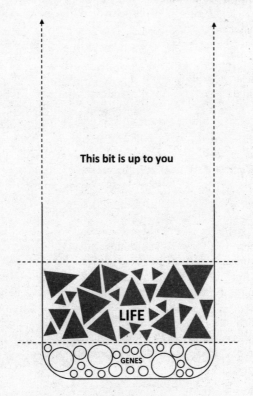

This bit is up to you

LIFE

GENES

Then we need **the things that are special to us**. I couldn't live without sport – doing and watching – or music – doing and listening. What is your equivalent? Put it in there.

Your jam jar doesn't need to be static. Since designing mine above, we have a new dog, Skye, and she would definitely be an extension all of her own now.

The jam jar can be as big or as small as you like, provided you are happy with the content of those extensions, and then build them into your life and keep checking that you are taking care of them. Ever since I have been consciously trying to do this, I have in the main felt better and happier. The plunges still come. But my jam jar not only helps me stave them off, it has given me the tools to deal with them when the dark cloud is heading towards me. I hope yours helps you too.

INDEX

INDEX

INDEX

INDEX

INDEX

INDEX

INDEX

INDEX

INDEX